How to find health

Step 4
The Benefits of Natural Diet

Diego Pagani

ISBN-13: 978-1727143331
ISBN-10: 1727143337

English translation by Martina Bassi

DEDICATION
This book is dedicated to you.

I want to thank <u>Claudio Nicolig</u> for his fundamental support for the drafting of this text, without which the most scientific part would not have been so detailed and thorough.
Thanks also to <u>Lorenza Lullo</u> for introducing me to the world of food and for her help and support during the writing of the book.

Index

DISCLAMER

1 ABOUT THE AUTHOR: DIEGO PAGANI

I was born lucky; I had a happy childhood. I was loved and cared for in the best possible way by my parents, in addition to having the affection of all four grandparents. Aside from having had my tonsils out as a child, I have always had excellent health; to my great good fortune, I have never had to experience what it means to be really sick. During adolescence, my relationship with disease was non-existent. In consequence, I was not disturbed by the idea of sickness, and the idea even intrigued me a little. Over time, I experience the deaths one by one of my grandparents. Like any ordinary person, I have suffered a lot, but this, I thought, was normal. Like most people who have arrived at a certain age, I conceived of the emergence of diseases that lead to death as a natural consequence of life. How wrong I was!

Unfortunately, years later, my mother, who was just over forty, was hit by breast cancer, to which the "perfect modern medical science" opted for chemotherapy and removal of the breast. But as is so often the case with doctors, they could not save her life, but only lengthen it briefly. A few years after the operation, her breast cancer recurred in a more serious form, in the liver. Despite months of "cures" still based on chemotherapy, she died, after having first suffered terribly and been physically devastated. Nobody, but nobody, had warned my mother that proper diet could have saved her life. Today, in light of what I have learned, I am convinced that if my mother had changed her diet from the moment she was first diagnosed with breast cancer and later liver cancer, she would still be here and certainly would have helped me write this book.

Despite the death of my mother, my confidence in Western medicine was still unchanged and my ignorance on nutrition continued. I had not even remotely begun to suspect that such physical disruption could have been caused by unhealthy eating habits. Mistaken beliefs about nutrition can be passed down from mother to daughter with all good intentions, allowing a choice of foods that are apparently healthy, but in the long run, kill!

Apart from the family drama for me and my father, at the time I did not have any great curiosity in this terrible disease, not because it did not interest me as a result of killing my mother, but because I still had confidence in doctors and in "progress." Accordingly, both during the illness and after, I felt sure that the care and the methods applied had been the best possible, but, unfortunately, given the severity of the disease, it was impossible to do anything else.

A few years ago my father was diagnosed with throat cancer and underwent an operation. To my great thankfulness, he is now alive and has almost fully recovered. Also on this occasion, in addition to the sorrow one naturally feels at the illness of a loved one, I was not interested in the technical aspect of the disease because, once again, I assumed that the professional preparation of the doctors (favored by all these years of scientific research) was the only useful solution to help my father.

Sure, he smoked, and the onset of cancer was certainly encouraged by this undesirable habit, but now I realize that smoking was not the only cause and, probably, without that drawback, he could have healed without the need to undergo such a devastating surgery. While it is true that the operation saved him, but at the same time, it left him in a much debilitated condition, while leaving him in worse shape than before the surgery, plus brought him years of suffering that was certainly avoidable.

Today, in light of the information that I have since gained, I realize that if my father (in addition to giving up smoking) had changed his diet to one of good nutrition, his health might still be good. To some degree, I feel a little responsible for both the death of my mother and the great suffering that my father has experienced. Of course, I know I was not at fault for these events, but I realize that most of the information that I have collected over the last few years has in fact been available for many decades, perhaps more. This makes me think that if I had known sooner, I could have changed the course of events.

But this did not happen. Therefore, I hope with my books to help those who are still shrouded in the fog of ignorance and give you the means to find your way to thrive and especially to avoid seeing those you love fall ill needlessly and to undergo similar rounds of terrible suffering. In my first 40 years I never thought about my health, feeling myself to be normally healthy and in excellent health. Nutrition and especially its relationship with disease was not a topic of interest for me; I did not care about the topic and maybe I did not believe such a discussion was worthwhile, either. Left to my own devices, I was not particularly interested in various types of diets. I only knew the term "vegetarian" and I had never even heard the word "vegan." In my ignorance, the correlation between health and food was for me a completely unknown argument.

Until the age of forty years, I was nourished in the "traditional" way, namely eating a bit of everything—meat, fish, pasta, bread, rice, salads, fruit, etc. The only food that I never ate was cheese, not for dietary reasons, but just because I never liked it (thankfully). I have a normal physique, tending to slender. I am tall, at 1.80 meters and weighing 70 kilograms, and I've never been a big "glutton." I do not deny having spent evenings at restaurants enjoying the taste of some of my favorite foods, but I have always eaten just to eat; I ate just because "I needed to" take in nourishment. My relationship with food has definitely helped me change my eating habits toward the natural diet without having to regret my old eating habits; I repeat, I'm lucky.

In recent years, I have devoted my energy almost entirely to the study of nutrition and the effects it has on health. I have no medical training; I am not a doctor and I have not used expensive equipment. My only weapon has been a willingness to study and to gather information and collect many testimonies over the years from many people. Of course, I can speak from personal experience, because I have been able to carefully analyze the significant effects that a change has had on me, and on the people close to me. I consider myself a guinea pig, but a guinea pig lucky and happy to have discovered many truths!

I am convinced that, in this case, not being a doctor has helped me because I realized that too much knowledge (not always exact and often driven by economic interests) can easily create preconceptions. My initial ignorance allowed me to observe and experiment with my new frugivorous diet, observing events from a perspective completely absent from prejudice. My choice would appear to be unconscious and perhaps it was, but in addition to having perceived the sensation of being right, while I proceeded to what I was pursuing, my increasingly deepening studies assured me day after day that I was on the right path.

2 OLD AGE DOESN'T EXIST

Despite the common beliefs, the third age can be lived in full serenity, in excellent health, without stress and also with satisfying emotional relationships. If you have lived long enough to be identified as "old people" do not worry because rejuvenation is possible; a healthy and balanced life, full of activity, full of joy of life is within everyone's reach. The so-called third age can be lived in full health, it depends only on your future choices, especially the food choices.

In the culture of the peoples of the whole world, old age has always been considered an irreversible process that accompanies man through heavy periods; I think instead that thanks to all the experiences accumulated in the years lived, the third age should be the most interesting and productive period of the life of each of us.

Unfortunately, most of today's elders navigate between a disease and the other, spends their days bouncing between the doctor and the laboratory for analysis, enters and exits the hospitals and does nothing but talk to friends and relatives of their diseases .

It is now considered normal that the elderly live with their illnesses and few are aware that the age in which we enter this "club" of perennial sick patients is always lower.

The various more or less serious diseases, erroneously attributable to old age, prevent those who have been lucky enough to live longer to enjoy the last years as they would like.

It saddens us to think of pensioners who, after working for years only to obtain a certain economic stability, now that they could enjoy life, are, because of the wear and tear of the body, forced to give up a happy and full of activity existence.

The typical diseases of old age should not actually exist. Conventional medicine today seeks to alleviate only its symptoms: examination after examination, pill after pill, surgery after surgery and day after day, the elderly is unknowingly dragged by the system into an unseemly path that will accompany him until the day of his departure.

Authoritative scientific research shows that animals have an average life that is seven times longer than they take to develop completely.

Man reaches his physical development at about twenty years old, so it is easy to calculate that his biological age should be about one hundred forty years old. Today the society sees in a ninety-year-old man, shriveled and senile, an extraordinary event to celebrate, perceiving as if he were some kind of miracle of nature.

If the whole of mankind were more prepared in matters of nutrition, people would not only live much longer, but would live better and healthier, moreover, by not requiring more care, they would not burden the state monetary budgets, so that the whole community would be richer also economically.

After birth, growth and development, we reach maturity and finally death: this is the natural path of every living being. As we can see, old age is not mentioned because it is not necessary for the completion of the life cycle.

Death can be achieved without necessarily going through a period of physical and mental decadence; the human being should naturally turn off in his bed without suffering and sadness, showing gratitude and satisfaction for having lived a wonderful life.

Animals in nature do not age accumulating diseases of all kinds, they simply switch off when their time comes.

Grouping all the sick people of a certain age, calling them "old" means normalising a situation that should instead be an exception: the adjective "old" should refer only to the time since the birth of an individual, however, this term is today used to define a state of health; in this way it is assumed that an old man must be ill.

It must be clear in mind that old age is a disease that does not exist.

Humanity has come to accept this state of decadence. Most people wait for old age without thinking about conserving their health: for the rest of their lives they are passively waiting for the infirmities to arrive and then consider themselves "finally" old.

The official science not knowing how to solve the general decay that affects everyone, considers it an irreversible and non-pathological state. Medicine, without analyzing the real causes, declares that at some point in life, the cells, the glands, the organs slow down their activities and that the various pathologies that affect us are nothing more than natural symptoms of old age.

It is not so, let's see why: the intoxication of the body caused by wrong feeding starts from early childhood, until you are in the first phase of life (the effects of waste and toxins usually do not cause immediate damage); it is only with the passing of the years that the continuous accumulation of these poisons, day after day, becomes a cause of obstruction and constipation for the whole organism, thus giving rise to the first signs of senility: weakness, lower performance, worn out appearance, decreased hearing, wrinkles, baldness, white hair, loss of vision, memory and weakened reflections, impotence, rheumatism, etc. they are not symptoms of old age, but of too many toxins accumulated over the years!

The pathological condition that is found in older people, then, is nothing but the progressive intoxication caused by the consumption of wrong foods: this is the only cause that causes all the symptoms classified as "diseases of old age".

When a diet based on fruit is used, blood circulation benefits, peripheral ramifications of blood vessels and lymphatic vessels are released from mucus and toxins, making each capillary able to adequately feed all the cells, so the wrinkles progressively they will withdraw, the skin will return elastic, sight and hearing will improve, the white hair will slowly disappear and the ailments will gradually reduce.

Wrinkles and withered skin are a sign of deep dehydration caused by the lack of organic water. In a truly nourished body, consequently hydrated and free from accumulation of waste, the skin cells are continuously sprayed with blood which, flowing vigorously, carries all the necessary nutrients, making the skin from head to toe velvety, elastic, smooth and bright.

To start the rejuvenation process, the body will need time and this will depend on the degree of personal intoxication, therefore on the level of obstruction of the organism: the more the person who intends to rejuvenate is overweight or too intoxicated by waste and poisons, the longer it will be its purification path. Only by virtue of the correct choice of food, it will be possible to reach a level of purification that will allow the first signs of rejuvenation to appear.

Today's medical science through its methods is not able to rejuvenate and the administration of drugs, in fact, increases the amount of poisons inside the body that adding to the already existing waste, accelerates the aging process, but to heal from old age as you have seen it is possible and feasible in a completely natural way.

Cosmetic surgery is just an unnatural and harmful palliative, it only serves to make young people appear intoxicated and sick, it only serves to make people look like what they really are not.

What we mean is a real state of youth, a condition of seniority that in addition to showing a more youthful appearance, includes a well-being on all fronts, among which an excellent mental lucidity strengthened by a strong psychological balance.

If you want to live, if you are rich in willpower, trust in nature and in the perfect machine that is your body, simply choose to follow with perseverance a diet that can help you achieve a perfect condition. So you can continue to live escaping all the ailments and pains of those who instead choose to continue with self-destructive food habits. Remember that old age is nothing but an advanced intoxication, the choice of how to live your last years is only in "your hands".

3 THE NATURAL DIET FOR MEN

Hair loss

In men the state of the hair is one of the major parameters to assess the general state of health, in fact the poisonous waste resulting from a pleasure feeding, over the years accumulate in the body up to cause even hair loss.

In recent decades, more and more young people are bald, a symptom that reveals a body encumbered with poisons. Unfortunately, a good part of modern youth shows a poor state of health that anticipates the advent of future diseases and infirmities, normally found only in people of advanced age. The nicotine in cigarettes, the uric acid generated by the consumption of animal products, the acetic acid caused by the consumption of refined foods and sweets, the muriatic acid originating from the consumption of coffee and tea and the carbonic acid produced by consumption of gassed drinks, they are the real architects that trigger the physical reaction responsible for baldness.

As you have already read at the beginning of this book, our body to neutralize excess acids, uses minerals such as calcium, sodium, potassium, magnesium and zinc, all substances that should be taken through proper nutrition.

When this does not happen or is not enough, these minerals are subtracted from the stocks previously accumulated in the body. Fortunately, the human body contains stocks of mineral substances in the bones, teeth, nails, hair and scalp, and it is precisely here that is the cause of premature loss of hair: when the acidity of the body is so high that not even the minerals in the blood are able to neutralize it, to protect teeth and bones, the body initially takes from the scalp the minerals necessary to neutralize the acids. In this case the use of this mineral reserve is vital, but this means depriving the scalp of its minerals, and after having been "demineralized" it will no longer be able to preserve the hair.

Excess sport is another factor that causes hair loss because it favors the formation of lactic acid which, if produced in excessive quantities, becomes a poison for the whole organism. This creates the same situation as before, the excess of lactic acid is removed with the same procedure by which the other acids present in the body are eliminated, that is to say, by plundering the mineral stockpiles.

Any sporting activity, especially when intense or practiced at a professional level, should always be carried out in conjunction with a natural diet, rich in organic mineral salts that help keep the level of lactic acid low even during prolonged physical exertion. The baldness therefore, will be more marked the more serious the state of intoxication of the person.

Even those who have an enviable head of air have their problems, the most annoying and obvious of which is dandruff. The body, in fact, getting rid of toxins, even through the scalp, often produces hated dandruff. However, there is good news for both "peeled" and "hairy man": a healthy and purifying diet is capable even after a few months, first to definitively make disappear any trace of dandruff, then to trigger a slow but constant regrowth of hair.

Here I would like to add a personal note, before changing diet, while still having all the hair I have always noticed a fair presence of dandruff and I was slowly losing some hair.

I can absolutely confirm that after only a few months of fruitarian nutrition, not only there was no more traces of dandruff but also my hair "miraculously" grew back, where they were thinning a bit too much. I also noticed that my few white hairs are progressively disappearing. If you eat fruit you will always have loads of hair and the original color, otherwise you can always resort to lotions, dyes, transplants or wigs.

Impotence

Yes, the traditional diet now followed around the globe based on pasta, bread, pizza, meat, milk, eggs, sweets, coffee, cigarettes, alcohol, etc., is also a cause of impotence.

In a body obstructed by slag, poisons and toxins, over the years even the veins that carry blood to the penis can occlude: such obstructions of the arterial walls prevent the blood from reaching the *corpus cavernosum* in sufficient quantity and pressure to inflate them until rigidity, thus compromising erection.

With the right nutrition the arteries and the *corpus cavernosum* of the penis will be reordered helping the blood, also cleaned and fluidised, to flow better facilitating the erection.

As known, there are today some stratagems that allow you to drink, smoke and eat in an inconsiderate way while continuing to carry out "interesting" activities.

Everyone knows the "magic pills" on sale today, which promise miracles and burning nights, but as well known they are very dangerous: some of the side effects mainly concern the function of the heart, causing arrhythmias and cardiovascular problems. It is useless and dangerous to follow easy shortcuts using products that, with the intent to provide certain advantages, cause enormous damage to the rest of the body.

Only nature can help the body to restore all its functions in a definitive way and without contraindications, because it is the only one that can "straighten" what the man with his stupidity has compromised.

Musculature

Many believe that to develop good muscles it is necessary to eat with very protein foods; eating large quantities of meat seems to be the only solution to obtain a muscular body, but who says it?

As already explained, proteins are contained even in vegetables more than enough to obtain a tonic and muscular body, even the strongest and most powerful mammals such as gorillas, elephants and bulls, are robust and powerful even though they eat only raw vegetables. Misinformation, prejudices and wrong advice, even if given in good faith, are all factors that induce "civilized" humanity to not understand that the same power that makes the gorillas strong and robust can lead man (of frugivorous nature too) to the same results.

Muscles are developed and maintained simply by using them in a job that requires physical effort or through sporting activities that are not necessarily heavy.

The natural diet allows to achieve, in terms of musculature, results far superior to the classic omnivorous diet. In addition, the muscles that are obtained by feeding properly are not fake and inflated by water retention as those of whom feed on animals. The muscles of all the fruitarians who practice a little sport seem more tapered, much stronger and more resistant; for these reasons, sportsmen, even professionals, who eat only with vegetables and lots of fruit, easily obtain better performances than their "carnivorous" colleagues.

In many, even if they are lucky enough to be aware of the natural diet, they do not feel like changing their lifestyle. Food tastes, even if they are wrong, are difficult to remove, especially when they are constantly supported by deceptive advertising that drives everyone to think the same way or, as we believe, not to think at all.

"But how? Everyone eats meat, so it means is good! "

Take for example a great meat eater like the Hollywood star John Wayne, known all over the world and still considered by many to be an example of masculinity. This famous actor has been a model followed by several generations of men and boys, who to imitate their manhood have imitated his style of food by increasing even the quantities, swallowing pounds of meat, drinking rivers of beer and smoking mountains of cigarettes. Still, many follow that example only to show themselves and others to be "*true man or hard man*" they have unfortunately grown with this image and continue to perceive it as positive.

Unfortunately, like many of his admirers, John Wayne died at the age of seventy-two because of one of the most common tumors, imputed to the consumption of meat: stomach cancer.

The natural diet improves the character and amplifies the sensitivity towards all living beings, however some men are afraid of becoming too sensitive, thus believing to lose their masculinity; in some cultures the idea still prevails that man must be "macho" hard and insensitive. In reality, both children and women greatly appreciate sensitivity in a man, but rather increase in them the perception of "real man".

It is time for masculinity to change, to definitely increase muscle and keep fit by doing physical activity is absolutely right and recommended, but let's not forget that increasing your sensitivity will also improve interpersonal relationships and certainly this will be appreciated by all those around us. It is not necessary to feed on dead animals, moreover killed by others, to demonstrate their virility.

Choosing to feed in a healthy way is often perceived as a drastic and difficult change of habits, so this choice will be an example for all those who know you: you will demonstrate a strong, independent and impervious character to mass thinking.

In the last decades more and more families have lost the male figure, men and boys die because of heart attack, cancer, diabetes, etc. It is not only the misfortune of the departure to tear the family, it is also the painful situation during the illness to upset the lives of their loved ones.

I believe that no man would want to be a burden on his family, especially because of health problems due to personal wrong choices: the amputation of a leg, sexual impotence and the infirmity that many diseases cause, upset not only the existence of those affected, but also of the people around him.

A "fat and bald" man who is in a hospital room attached to tubes is not synonymous with masculinity; an intelligent man should have the courage to think about his own health, not only for himself, but also for his loved ones, his wife and especially his children.

4 THE NATURAL DIET FOR WOMEN

*Since I am not a woman, I have written this chapter on the indica-
tions of Lorenza Lullo, who has adopted
the natural diet as well.*

Beauty

If women would discover the existence of a secret
method that can always keep them young, beautiful and
in perfect health, they certainly would do anything to get
it.

Through exclusively a fruit-only diet, you can obtain the
true long-life elixir that will give you beauty and youth
in a totally natural, economical way, without using various creams and lotions, without taking supplements or
herbal products and without the need to resort to cosmetic surgery.

Day after day and with patience, a frugivorous diet will
improve not only your psychological and healthful appearance, but also the aesthetic one, making you perfect
as you are destined to be.

The skin of the young will remain perfect for a long time
or, in case of imperfections such as acne, dryness or

greasy epidermis, it will be able to heal and regenerate completely.

The first results that will be noticed will be luminous, voluminous hair, smoother and above all soft and hydrated without the use of balms; the hair will keep clean longer, white hair will disappear, while the regrowth will be abundant and of the original color. The nails will become strong, smooth, shiny and without imperfections.

Then with perseverance and confidence, on the face of older women, wrinkles will be drastically attenuated as if by magic and the skin will return elastic, hydrated and silky giving the face brightness and firmness. Fruit is the food that helps the body to hydrate the cells more deeply, so it is the only one able to facilitate the disappearance of these symptoms of deep dehydration.

Aesthetic defects such as eye bags, dark circles, dark spots, blotches, mole, are mainly caused by the consumption of animal products and will vanish totally because they are only symptoms of dysfunctions that the body wants to signal making them evident especially on the face.

As you have read by reading the chapter that illustrates the phenomenon of leukocytosis, if you will eat only raw food, the amount of white blood cells will be reduced to the advantage of red blood cells: your face will reflect a new total well-being through a beautiful rosy color, while the lips will take a natural red color making the use of make-up and lipstick unnecessary.

Thanks to the cleaned blood, even the tanning will be more intense and uniform, a long exposure to the sun will no longer be necessary and the golden color will appear more quickly making the use of tanning creams useless.

About creams, we remind you that sun protectors and tanning should not be used because they considerably slow down the natural transpiration of the skin, inhibiting the absorption of the ultraviolet rays essential for the body.

Know that 90% of sunscreens contain octylmethoxycinnamate, a toxic chemical that, ironically, doubles the effects of its own toxicity when exposed to sunlight. These products also impede the proper functioning of the glands that secrete protective substances: it is true that they allow prolonged exposure to the sun, but since they only protect the first superficial layer of the skin, the underlying connective tissue could be permanently damaged causing the premature aging of the whole body.

The redness of skin that manifests itself during prolonged exposure to the sun is a warning that nature adopts to warn us that the time has come to take shelter in the shade.

In addition to sunscreens, even all cosmetic products should be avoided because most are a real poison; while they only give a temporary relief, at the same time they cause enormous damage to the whole body. When the various creams are applied, about 60% of the petroleum-derived chemicals, which many are composed, will be absorbed through the pores of the skin, to finish up accumulated in the liver and kidneys: it is exactly as if you would ingest all the toxic substances present in cosmetics. Oils, lotions and deodorants also have the disadvantage of occluding the pores of the skin preventing the natural transpiration and leakage of the slag, as naturally should happen because the surface of the skin, as previously written, is one of the excretory organs for the elimination of toxins. Another advantage offered by our nutrition is the effect that is found on the sweating that will be reduced and odorless making any type of deodorant useless.

Remember that the skin hydrates and nourishes itself exclusively from the inside through organic water and vitamins.

Lorenza says: *"I know it well, because since I was born I suffered from a severe form of eczema extended all over my body: I applied tons of creams of every kind without receiving absolutely any benefit. Only now I understood that with creams and cortisone, I did nothing but reintroduce daily the waste that my body was trying to eliminate through the skin.*

Since I totally changed my diet, both asthma and eczema have completely disappeared leaving me a perfect skin without having to use absolutely any moisturizer.

If you are still forced to use moisturizers and cosmetics, I recommend at least to choose certified organic ones, they are certainly less invasive.

The animal products and all vegetable fats such as oils and margarines, are the cause of the reduction of blood circulation and one of the negative effects is the appearance of capillaries, an anti-aesthetic consequence also easily eliminated by following our diet: me too, I saw my capillary disappear from my legs."

A deeply cleansed body will no longer present those annoying symptoms such as swollen legs and ankles, the calves and knees will become slimmer, developing a more harmonious profile and, thanks to the disappearance of any cellulite, will acquire form and sensuality.

Women who do not boast a great décolleté will see their breasts increase by a size, while those with a prosperous breasts will notice a remarkable firming.

The natural diet will give a well-defined and feminine harmonious body with the right bends, the flat abdomen, the regenerated connective tissue and the more toned musculature.

Do not you think that all this is a great secret of beauty? It is no coincidence that more and more Hollywood actresses, persuaded by the power of fruit, are adopting the natural diet.

Menstruation

Although manifesting in the majority of women, menstruation is never a sign of good health, but represents an event closely related to your degree of intoxication. Any woman if she could eliminate the annoying and often painful menstrual cycle, would do so willingly. The monthly appearance is not a sign of health since menstruation is just one way the body gets rid of poisons and toxins accumulated between one cycle and another; in women who feed mainly on high-protein foods like meat, fish, eggs, milk and cheese, the flow is often very intense and accompanied by severe pain

Premenstrual syndrome with its symptoms of depression, nervousness, irritability, migraine, swelling, etc., is also absolutely determined by what it's eaten; it is customary to believe that during the premenstrual period, breast pain is normal, while the cause is due to intestinal inflammation caused by the intake of cereals such as rice, bread, pasta, flour and starches such as potatoes and corn.

Between one flow and the other, the woman does not metabolize the acidifying products and the waste, but accumulates them in the blood, in the lymph and in the case of pregnancy also in the placenta, so, until the day of menstruation, the acidity levels will increase reaching a concentration such as to create the disorders commonly called "premenstrual syndrome".

When the accumulation of acids reaches the highest level, the belly and the legs as the whole body, will swell with water (edema) to dilute the acids and the waste present: with the arrival of menstruation, it will start the procedure that leads to the expulsion of waste and poisons with the relative disappearance of all symptoms.

Contrary to a high protein diet, a diet based on raw fruits and vegetables, purifies the body by relieving it of waste and poisons, which as we have seen are the cause of menstruation, the menstrual flow can be shorter, lighter and painless.

Well, it seems incredible, but a natural way to gradually eliminate menstruation exists. With a healthy diet, the body thus cleaned will gradually reduce the flow until the disappearance of pain and premenstrual syndrome.

Only with a natural diet based exclusively on fruit consumption one can obtain such a pure body till menstruation is an old memory.

Normally, menstruation occurs about once a month to ensure that the body remains clean enough in anticipation of an imminent conception. It was discovered that it is thanks to this phase of "cleaning up" that statistically women live about ten years more than men.

If we consider the days that accompany menstruation as not fertile, it will be obvious that in the absence of flow, these days will return to be potentially fertile. Ovulation in women can occur without menstruation and, unlike common thinking, these two processes are completely independent of each other.

Estrogens are the sex hormones responsible for female characteristics such as breast, silhouette and the distribution of fat in the body; these hormones are formed at the level of adipose tissue through a specific enzyme: aromatase. Thanks to the lipids a conversion occurs in the adrenal glands: the aromatase converts the androgens that are present in these glands into estrogens. However, several causes can lead to an inappropriate increase in estrogen hormones: the intake of the contraceptive pill and / or drugs, the consumption of all types of animal products (including butter, milk, eggs and all fats of animal origin), fried food , sweets and fats extracted or concentrated also of vegetable origin (extra virgin olive oil, seed oil, margarine, linseed oil, etc.). All these foods should be avoided because they cause excessive estrogen production.

The modern woman who lives in the so-called "advanced civilization" has in her body an excessive quantity of estrogen hormones just because of a wrong diet. To bring these hormones back to ideal levels, it will be necessary to categorically eliminate the intake of animal fats, but it would be also preferable to reduce the amount of fats of plant origin as much as possible: this will result in a noticeable drop in estrogen blood levels.

All vegetable foods, having a high fiber content, help the body to expel excess estrogens; the estrogens through the liver are brought from the bloodstream to the digestive tract where they will be retained by the fruit and vegetable fiber, to be then carried with them to the expulsion.

We believe it is very important to point out that, without the help of an adequate amount of fiber, estrogens would remain in circulation and then reabsorbed by the blood system. Recall that an excessive number of estrogens in the body can cause various interferences on the menstrual process.

Now it seems that many people know that the use of the contraceptive pill is harmful, and this is true because its use causes a reduced menstrual flow and an artificial leak, triggered just by the hormones introduced with it. For this reason, the body will no longer be able to fulfill the expulsion of poisons as naturally would occur during menstruation and will have negative consequences such as stagnation of poisons, water, cellulite, loss of hair, skin problems, loss of libido, migraines and, moreover, the body, holding the liquids to dilute the accumulated toxic acids, among which the hormones of the pill itself, will increase in weight.

In conclusion we can state that the menstrual cycle is not the cause, but the effect of the intoxication of one's own body.

Personally I can say that my cycle is now particularly reduced without presenting the previous pains and the related premenstrual syndrome. I am convinced that in some time I will reach what would be a dream for me, to be totally free from the cycle.

Maternity

It is important to understand how during pregnancy, acids and waste continue to accumulate in the body and that, as we have already written, even the placenta filling itself with these poisons could create damage to the unborn child, so the quality of nourishment that will receive from the mother during gestation will be essential to avoid possible health problems for the child.

If the mother during the maternity will not give up the animal products and will not feed with fruit in abundance, various complications could arise such as nausea, headache, hair loss, fall of teeth, hemorrhoids, etc.: such symptoms reveal that during the absence of menstruation, the organism still has the need to expel its poisons.

Symptoms of detoxification, followed by light illnesses due to a sudden variation in diet, are the reasons why it is not advisable to change diet *during pregnancy or breastfeeding*, the ideal would be to implement a natural diet based on only fruit at least six months before conception. If man also followed a correct diet, he would favor the procreation of a perfect creature, a child who never cries, always joyful and healthy. The dream of every parent, a result easily obtainable if you want to change the style of food nourishing yourself in the right way.

From the embryonic stage today's children are over-fed and intoxicated, giving the mother a difficult and painful delivery: there is no valid reason why the expectant mother should feed twice as much as normal, it's enough to increase the intake of natural and organic sweets: fresh fruit and dried fruit.

The first cause of death in children under three years of life is due to breathing problems. The respiratory syndrome would seem to be caused by the consumption of milk, cheese and various dairy products, which women supplement their diet during pregnancy. If during pregnancy, the new mother encouraged by inadequate and confused advice, will continue to feed with dairy products, will provide significant damage to the unborn child. In recent years a very close correlation has been discovered between the protein comes in the form of a dense and thick liquid and it is found in huge quantities inside the lungs of infants affected by respiratory problems and died prematurely and taking dairy products during pregnancy.

Because of this, newborns of mothers who feed on dairy products during pregnancy are often subjected to the mechanical aspiration of mucus that clogs their respiratory tract; this procedure is not necessary for children born to mothers who did not take dairy products during gestation.

Once again, the responsibility of milk products is evident and their danger does not only manifest itself at the time of birth, but brings consequences for the whole life of the child in the form of serious diseases, among which the asthma is an example among the most annoying and common.

Therefore, during pregnancy, it is absolutely vital to pay more attention to food, fruit and vegetables are foods that feed in the most correct way both mother and child.

Menopause

During the menopause, the purification method resulting from menstruation is missing, so if you do not promptly intervene with a proper diet, all the acids and poisons will accumulate in the body causing some typical male health problems: fat in the abdomen, loss of hair, excessive sweating preceded by the typical hot flashes. The menopause is technically a progressive deterioration of specific glands that attacked by acids, atrophy, making them unable to help the mechanism for the production of estrogen hormones, hormones that are crucial for female fertility.

Unfortunately, modern women, due to an increasingly incorrect diet based on animal products, preserved foods, frozen foods, coffee, dairy products, etc., have their glands more and more acid and consequently the system interrupts early the production of estrogens.

It can therefore be said that in a body cleaned of acids and toxins, the aforementioned glands not atrophying will be able to do their job and consequently the "pure" woman will be really young and fertile for many more years.

5 THE NATURAL DIET FOR CHILDREN

Parents have a huge responsibility towards their children, they are the "creators" of future adults and therefore should be able to give them the best education.

In my opinion, a fundamental lesson that a good and careful parent should transmit to their children, is precisely about nutrition, since it will depend the future of those who are growing up; as we shall see, the right food choice will not only affect the state of health, but also the emotional and psychological one.

I am well aware that parenting is not easy, even in the field of nutrition there are too many contradictory information that creates confusion. Those parents who want to follow a natural lifestyle, far away and independent of common thinking, are often faced with great difficulties, because they are bewildered by advice or even directives that come from the "experts" of the standard medical-nutritional system. Vaccines are an example. In this text I not cover this thorny topic because it is not part of the food discourse, but I advise you to inform yourself well, online you can find many sites where are exposed the various consequences, even serious, that the vaccines can cause especially to the most little ones.

So, apart from the medical advice and the obligatory (fortunately avoidable today) of having to vaccinate their children, exposing them to potential dangerous consequences, you must also be on guard regarding the various advice in the food field that doctors, pediatricians, nutritionists, friends, parents, grandparents and relatives give you daily (even if in good faith), with the intent, according to them, to make your children grow well.

Both multinational food companies and pharmaceutical companies sell an enormous amount of industrially produced denatured food every day which, as we have seen in other chapters, are harmful to the health of everyone. Some of these products have been created just for the little ones. Your children are the first victims of these poisons, disguised as food presented in beautiful packaging on which there are captivating photographs and cunning descriptions in which it refers, even, to non-existent nutritional or healthy properties.

While selling their merchandise, multinational food through advertising and improper messages, persist in hammering baby consumers, who attracted and intrigued by the spots seen on TV, cannot do nothing but insistently ask their parents such deleterious "foods".

Is often difficult for parents and grandparents not to please the children's requests, but here we are not talking about harmless toys, here we are discussing the health and future of your children.

Foods like hamburgers, hot dogs, crisps, pizzas, snacks, chocolate, ice creams, sweets and sodas, are just harmful and denatured fillers that every child, if instructed correctly, could and should avoid. Children should realize as soon as possible how important it is to be responsible for their own health. This is fundamental both for their growth and for their future, remembering that low quality food develops low quality men.

Overly protein diets based on meat, eggs and cow's milk that children have been fed since childhood are imposed with extreme ignorance by the world pediatric system. In small and unaware creatures, this diet facilitates the emergence of diseases and sufferings that otherwise would not know. In fact, children have an innate sense that leads them instinctively to reject meat.

A famous American pediatrician dr. Robert Mendelsohn, realized the progress of modern pediatrics and often repeated: "*Is your baby well? Do not go to the pediatrician, he will get sick of it. Is he sick? Do not go to the pediatrician, it would aggravate him. Did you go there? Do exactly the opposite of what he told you and you will do a great favor to your little child*".

The natural expectation of life of man should be around one hundred and forty years but because of the food errors perpetuated since childhood, if lucky he will not be able to live beyond ninety. Not only that: you will probably reach this miserable goal struggling among numerous illnesses, which you will try to cure through the use of medicines or surgical interventions.

This will be the future of your children and it is your present. To avoid all this, living longer and above all in health, there is no choice but to pay close attention to your diet.

During childhood it is essential to choose the right diet because it is at this stage that the child grows and his character is formed; his health will depend on his diet, his development, his performance and his personality. Today, unfortunately, in children there is a double percentage of chronic diseases, compared to a few decades ago, while all children should be the living expression of health, vigor, joy and serenity.

If your child has symptoms like otitis, cough or cold, you are probably feeding him with cow's milk and derivatives; try to eliminate them and you will notice in your child, after an initial worsening due to the elimination of mucus, a noticeable improvement, until the total disappearance of all the symptoms, so you will spare your child useless troubles and sufferings. Do not think that otitis, sore throat, runny nose, "fat" cough and fever are normal and natural childhood diseases.

The fact that such nuisances and symptoms are present in almost all children means that almost all children feed badly.

Symptoms are reactions that the body puts in place to warn that something is not proceeding in the right way, but instead of paying attention to such signals, traditional medicine ignores them. Unfortunately, very often parents do not have the sensitivity or culture to recognize the reason for the appearance of various symptoms. Most of them ignore the fact that the only natural and harmless way to reverse the illness would be simply to immediately stop taking all the wrong foods, replacing them with healthy and natural products. It is not difficult to replace milk, ice cream, potato chips and various sweets with fruit, even in the form of juices and centrifuged, natural foods that children usually appreciate very much.

Personally, I happened several times to witness situations in which the children wanted fruit and, after eating it with taste and joy, strongly refused what the parents considered a healthy lunch based on meat or fish. I have seen children cry because they did not want to eat meat and parents insist to the extreme in wanting to swallow their children of such harmful food, thinking of doing them good.

How much ignorance on the part of the parents and how much truth hidden behind the whims of the little ones. If only once in a while would you listen to the signs of nature and the instincts of children not yet conditioned by this confused world, it would all be much simpler.

Medical science never seeks the causes of illness, but through drugs it seems only interested in suppressing its symptoms: in doing so it slows down the body's attempt to clean itself of excess waste, mucus and poisons, often leading to a progressive worsening of the diseases themselves.

The cause that determines all diseases is nutrition, a fact that is also valid for children, 98% of children have at least one predisposing factor for heart disease, 75% are overweight, 42% are found in the blood an intolerable cholesterol level, the cases of obese children are constantly increasing, while the main cause of juvenile death is cancer.

The latter data refer to the population of the United States of America which, thanks to the SAD (Standard

American Diet), holds the first place in the ranking of the worst-fed peoples; unfortunately also the rest of the world, Europe an Asia in the lead, is quickly reaching this sad record.

It is sad to think that it is not possible to rely on today's medical science to decrease the cases of cancer or other serious diseases that affect the children of the so-called welfare society every day, the only defense against such ailments can come only from ourselves and from our choices.

There is no valid reason why today continue to allow your children to feed themselves with foods that do not feed, that are died, deprived of their nutritional value, containing salt, sugar, animal fats and all the poisons that the food industry continues to produce.

Responsibility is in your hands, in your choices and in your desire to see your little ones grow up happy and healthy. To overlook with indifference on the subject of feeding, considering it marginal, proves to be the most serious attack against your health and your children.

I've read that some pediatricians have declared that a fat child can better withstand any ailments. I do not understand what the scientific basis is for affirming such a thing, fortunately most doctors are well aware of the problems and the consequences of being overweight.

In fact, in reality, there are no reasons to suggest that an obese child is really healthy, on the contrary there are clear evidence that they confirm that too much fat is harmful to the whole organism.

How many times have we heard from parents and especially grandparents that a child a bit plump is synonymous with well-being? A false myth probably resulting from anxieties born of having experienced the famine brought by the Second World War and the difficult period after.

Today, however, the situation is different, apart from some countries where you still die of hunger because of wars, in our society no one dies of hunger. Paradoxically, today we die just because of supercharging.

If a baby is fed as much as possible with breast milk, and soon after, with sweet fruit, he will have a much better chance of staying healthy. A frugivorous child who is contracting an illness (a rare hypothesis) will recover very quickly and naturally because his immune system, favored by a body free of toxins and poisons, will react more quickly and much more effectively than a child fed in the "traditional" way.

I can afford to say these things simply because we have met many fruitarian families, but also vegan and raw food, who do not even know what it means to have a sick child. The testimonies of happy parents of their natural food choices are everywhere, even online, just want to look for them.

With proper nutrition you can avoid your children all the suffering caused by diseases that will otherwise contract; today you have the opportunity to avoid your small headaches, stomach ache, acne, overweight, excess of anger and even emotional stress, all symptoms that affect most of today's children and adolescents.

A baby weaned with breast milk will surely have the instinct that will soon lead him to feed on fruit. Looking for a sweet taste, the child naturally shows that fructose is the natural basis of nutrition.

Fruit is the most biologically similar to mother's milk. However, be careful to avoid, at any cost, all industrial preparations such as homogenized fruit because they are rich in starches, sugar and various preservatives; therefore, as long as your child is not able to chew, it would be better to continue breastfeeding and gradually begin to make him taste grated or centrifuged fresh fruit.

Homogenized organic fruit in which a 100% fruit content is declared, without the addition of preservatives or other, could apparently be confused for excellent foods, but it is not so, in fact they are still boiled or pasteurized products, so they no longer have nothing in common with fresh fruit.

All packaged products such as baby food, ie corpse smoothies mixed with dead vegetables and various chemical compounds, should be avoided. Do not look for high-protein foods with the intent to grow your children well, remember that the mother's milk, which nature has made available to grow a newborn perfectly, has a protein content close to 1% in the normal of the child born after 9 months. Only in the case of premature birth, protein content in milk or colostrum is approaching 2%.

Children love fruit the same way they love sucking milk from their mother's breasts. In order to grow properly, children need to take high quality breast milk that contains all the necessary substances: if fed incorrectly or weaned prematurely, children may experience various problems. It is also essential that the mother during gestation and the breastfeeding period also feeds properly.

Therefore mothers, in addition to feeding with fruit of the best quality available (at least biological or better biodynamic), should be loved by the people around them, should rest all the time necessary and the last thing, but perhaps the most important, always keep a positive and serene attitude.

All mothers, if healthy and detoxified, always have plenty of milk because nature is never wrong. Those who have problems breast-feeding due to lack of milk can also find fault with this in their diet. The mother must have absolute confidence in herself and in nature, which sets and resolves everything to the best, one must only relax and keep in harmony with the experience of motherhood, allowing her body to produce all the milk that nature itself has predisposed for the growth of the child.

The mother's milk is really fundamental, for this reason the mother should continue to breastfeed until it is produced because the mother-newborn couple regulates itself.

It is no coincidence that even in this situation there is a perfect balance designed wonderfully by nature: the more the baby asks for nourishment by attaching himself to the breast, the more the mother will produce milk and this proves incontestably that the baby has the need to still feed breast milk. It may happen that the child's request for milk extends up to two years of age, this will be completely normal - the words WHO - Unicef says up to two years and even longer if mom and child want it - the feed for newborns mean much more than just taking food and only our unnatural society considers it correct to stop breastfeeding by replacing it with cow's milk.

It is not recommended to stop breastfeeding until the baby continues to request it because serious emotional imbalances can also arise; mothers who continue to breastfeed their baby for a long time, provide welfare both to their child and to society, helping to create better and healthier men.

There is no standard age for the baby in which to start including some fruit during weaning, each child will show the desire to try the fruit when he feels it necessary, probably ready after six months or after more than a year.

Try to offer the child a teaspoon of fresh fruit centrifuged between a feed and the other and observe his reaction, it will help you to understand if it is time for him to feed on fruit too; when the infant is able to chew, then it will be time for him to eat any kind of fruit.

Even for the little ones, the food change must proceed with caution, all the motivations of such prudence are exposed in the chapter of the transition. For children who are already accustomed to the classic diet and who are more than three years old, the transition to a plant or fruit-based diet is particularly delicate, you should not make the mistake of speeding up the change too much and you do not have to never force by force. Try to introduce more healthy food every day while decreasing the amount of harmful food, the transition must take place in a gentle way, so that the child gets used to new foods without realizing the changes.

It would be a great start to give the baby smoothies, centrifuged or fresh fruit juices for breakfast and snack; at the beginning of the meals you can increase the quantity of vegetables but if the child does not like it, you do not have to worry, you can give it the equivalent in fruit because the vegetables contain what also the fruit possesses.

If the baby often requires sweets or candies, it means that his body needs a greater supply of sugar and only the fructose contained in the fruit can adequately meet this need.

One day, when you see the little hands of your baby holding an apple, know that you have succeeded in making your child appreciate a food of immense value.

Sometimes, even on-line there are articles that try to illustrate what is the proper diet for human beings and often vegetarian, vegan and raw food diets are accused, by persuaded omnivorous, not to feed in sufficient way. From time to time, articles about vegan children with health problems appear on certain publications. None of these articles has ever, however, demonstrated in an accurate and scientific way the true cause of these presumed illnesses; so the writer of the article points the index on the choice of food, without even considering the type of disease, the family context and above all without analyzing the real nutrition that the unfortunate sick child has followed.

In modern society the image of "healthy child" is often depicted with images portraying overweight or too robust children, but this physical aspect does not represent in any way what should be a normal state of health.

It is true that children fed only fruit are usually leaner than their peers fed with sausages and pork, it is true that they have a smaller size when compared to their peers who adopt a diet full of chips and hamburgers, but that does not mean nothing. A slender body, especially in a child or adolescent, does not represent a negative characteristic at all; on the contrary: the lack of excess fat only proves to have a healthy body, free from waste and poisons.

The slower growth that occurs in children fed with plants or only with fruit is a positive trait. It is not a competition between those who grows before or after, but among those who grow up healthy or sick, small fruitarians have nothing to fear because with puberty their development will accelerate reaching both height and strength of their peers grown with cheese and mortadella. Nature has its time and, to do one thing well, it does not look at the calendar, is only goal is perfection, so be patient and trust, your children fed with the natural diet will have a perfect body as adults: any solid structure to be well built needs all the time necessary.

In nature, even gorillas, chimpanzees, orangutans, etc., show a slight build, but as you well know their adult development is clearly visible. There is no hurry in nature, everything happens when it is right for it to happen, the animals in nature reach the appropriate size only when they are able to provide for themselves.

In the meantime, as happens also for the human being, the little ones need to be looked after and protected. For example, in case of danger, small and light puppies should be carried in their parents' arms in safe places as quickly as possible. In this situation, the gorilla mother would have serious difficulties in saving her obese son, try to imagine the scene ...

No, fortunately it is an eventuality that does not exist in reality.

When a small child is held in his arms, he perceives beneficial human contact with his parents. Even in case of colic, take the baby up, it has an immediate calming effect: another case that shows how children should be well fed, but thin and light. Once again we notice the perfection that only nature possesses and that we can obtain only by following a life as much as possible in harmony with it.

Infants who are lucky enough to have a mother who feeds properly during breastfeeding, almost never suffer from colic and in case they are affected, they recover very quickly. The lucky children who will feed on fruit will not be victims of the classic diseases of childhood, they will be happy because they will grow following the design of nature, they will show good health, they will always live happy, they will always seek human contact and will be altruistic.

These qualities, as I have already written, will be presented to a greater extent if the mother, in addition to eating well, will have a peaceful pregnancy and will have the foresight to breastfeed the baby until it is necessary. I understand that a prolonged weaning for the mother, could be challenging, even for social or business reasons, but it will certainly be worth it. In order to have a better and more peaceful society, it is necessary to start with children and even before with newborns; in addition to the choice on proper nutrition, it is necessary to transmit to our children confidence in life, offering them absolute support without any reservation.

Children who will have the great fortune to be born of well-informed parents, will benefit from a privileged life, will have a balanced growth and will always enjoy good health, will be intelligent and sensitive people. Creativity, friendship, hope, optimism, love, correctness, integrity, harmony, perseverance, generosity, autonomy, serenity, wisdom, simplicity, kindness, they will all be your child's qualities.

6 TRANSITION TO THE NATURAL DIET

I am sure that at this point (if in addition to this book, you have also read the first three of the series "*How to find Health*") you have learned enough competence to discern between harmful foods and healthy foods, now you are able to choose the most appropriate food with which to feed yourself every day.

If you have understood correctly the importance of following a correct diet, you will certainly want to start a new life through natural food, but to start this food change you need to follow some important rules so that you can complete your journey in the more effective way. The rules I suggest you below are essential to reduce or eliminate any inconvenience that such a profound change could cause you.

My goal is to convey to all of you the awareness of how to achieve perfect health and this, as you will have understood, can only be achieved through proper nutrition.

When you stop taking acidifying foods, the body will eliminate the acids inside, the waste. These wastes are nothing but acids temporarily neutralized by substances recovered from the tissues. Our organism eliminates them according to the following steps: dissolution of the waste that returns to the circle; neutralisation of the same by means of products of plant origin; the so neutralized waste will be eliminated through the designated organs.

Nobody believes that speeding too much the transition between the two types of food can have benefits, indeed for most people, a change too sudden could cause significant disruption; this is why it is essential to follow a gradual process of change that could last from a few months to a few years.

This slow change, that we will call "*Transition Diet*".

Initially, even the best nourishment with the highest nutritional properties such as fruit, if consumed in the wrong way, could become harmful. For this reason you absolutely must go through the transition diet: this will allow you to "transit" gradually from the habit of feeding you with wrong foods, which produce the now known damages and discomforts, towards a natural diet comprising nutritious foods that, besides to promote health, meanwhile help to dissolve poisons.

The fruit, in fact, returns to the alkaline state and provides all the energy that the body requires, dissolves the poisons and helps the effective elimination of waste, even those returned in circulation.

This process is called detoxification, in other words, the natural elimination of waste accumulated in the body. The symptoms of detoxification will be different for each individual and could be revealed in a cyclical way, that is, in alternating phases. Some days will manifest intensely, while they may disappear for weeks and then reappear: all this will be normal, do not worry.

In some cases these symptoms could be completely absent, but in cases of elderly or obese people, detoxification may be more intense, so it is likely that it will manifest itself through those symptoms that cause greater discomfort. During the detox phase your body will use skin, mouth, lungs, intestines, kidneys in order to get rid of toxins and poisons accumulated meal after meal, day after day and year after year.

Have you ever thought about how many meals you have consumed since you came into the world?

In all likelihood you have begun to poison yourself as a child, so to cleanse your body, it will take time, be patient and trust.

Drowsiness, fatigue, loss of vitality, intestinal swelling, mild nausea, slight depression, sensitivity to light, cold, bad breath, pimples, skin rashes, more frequent bowel bleeding, gradual loss of weight, sore throat, fever, articular and muscular pain, are the classic symptoms of detoxification. A few other minor ailments, which in any case should not scare, although they can cause annoyances, are the precise signal that the body is eliminating toxic material; any other disturbance during the transitional diet is only caused by detoxification, so the only way to act during these phases is absolute rest; you should never take drugs because they would only increase the amount of poisons in the body by blocking the detoxification in place. We therefore note that what we normally call illness are only the organism's attempt to cleanse itself of poisons through the appropriate channels. When these symptoms manifest, it means that the body will be cleansed and everything will proceed in the right way. Proceed slowly through the transition diet, it is the correct method, but if this is not enough and signs of discomfort are manifested too strongly, then it will be good to slow down the transition eventually inserting incorrect foods, which will have the effect of slowing down detoxification making it more delicate, significantly reducing the annoying effects. To stand these disorders is the price to pay after years of binges that have deteriorated the body: you ate "food" of various kinds that maybe you thought healthy, now you have the opportunity to give your body the opportunity to cleanse and regenerate purifying and nurturing it, finally in the right way.

Immediately eliminating the so-called "junk foods" from the diet is the best way to start the transition, starting with the first purification phase.

Particular attention must be paid to nutritive pairings, avoiding incorrect food associations. You will then proceed to eliminate foods of animal origin, including all their derivatives and refined foods, replacing them with whole grains, legumes, cooked and raw vegetables, gradually adding more fruit to your diet, taking care to always take it away from meals. We will proceed in this way until we are fed only fruit, going through a period in which also raw vegetables, sprouts and seeds, will be part of the diet.

When we eat, we should be aware, not only of what we are taking, but also of the manner in which we perform one of the most important actions for the good of the whole organism, therefore for life itself. This being present and aware during meals is essential to allow our body to assimilate, as it should, all the nourishment it needs. Eating in a distracted way while doing something else, or worse, fast, even standing up, is an attitude that should be avoided.

During the transition, and even after, your meals will have to be consumed sitting, with calm and dedication, concentrating on the beneficial properties of what you are tasting; slow and persistent chewing helps assimilation of nutrients found in food, moreover, the predigesting effect that saliva puts in place against the ingested food, mixing with it, will significantly help digestion.

Another important aspect to keep in mind is that the body behaves differently in relation to the substances introduced during the day. Circadian rhythms help to better understand why during the various hours of the day the body behaves differently: from noon to eight pm you have the phase called of appropriation in which the food is taken and digested; from eight in the evening to four in the morning there is the assimilation phase, ie the absorption and use of food ingested food; from four in the morning to midday there is the phase of elimination in which the body gets rid of food residues and waste. This makes us understand how the habit of consuming a hearty breakfast in the morning is wrong because the food introduced during the elimination phase, has the negative effect of slowing it down causing the body a useless work supplement that causes tiredness and drowsiness, preventing effective elimination of accumulated toxins. Even eating too late in the evening over eight o'clock in the evening, has a bad effect because it upsets the biological rhythms of the body interfering with the assimilation phase postponing the work of the liver. This will lead to the symptoms of listlessness and fatigue that often arise upon awakening.

If as soon as you get up you feel the need to eat, then the fruit also taken in the form of juices or centrifuged is the only food that not only does not interfere with the elimination cycle, but rather, providing fibers and plenty of biological water, favors the process.

Let us now see in more detail how to proceed to put the transition diet into practice; as anticipated, the first step is to remove from the diet all those very harmful foods called "junk foods", in other words all stored foods, packaged foods, packaged chips, all packaged baked goods, sauces and condiments produced industrially, wine vinegar, energy drinks, carbonated drinks, all bottled or packaged fruit juices, white sugar, sweets, chocolate, cakes, ice creams, snacks, jams; coffee, wine, beer and alcohol in general; other foods to avoid are all frozen packaged foods.

We continue the transition diet while eliminating all incorrect associations between the various foods within the same meal. A meal is defined as food intake within an hour's time frame.

Protein foods such as meat, fish, chicken, eggs, dairy products, cured meats, legumes and nuts in general, should never be paired with each other (meat with eggs, omelette with ham, cheese with meat, etc.) and should never be combined neither with starches nor with cereals (chicken with potatoes, rice with beans, bread and ham, bread and cheese, pasta with meat sauce, pasta with beans, pasta with cheese, lasagne, cannelloni, etc.). The only food that goes perfectly with protein foods is raw and cooked vegetables, then a slice of meat, a plate of beans, a fried egg, a portion of cheese, a grilled fish, they all match exactly with a tasty mixed salad or a mix of boiled or better steamed vegetables.

Starches and cereals such as potatoes, rice, polenta, corn, pasta, bread and pizza, should never be taken during the same meal.

Therefore, the only food that combines with starches or cereals is once again vegetables, both cooked and raw, such as pasta with vegetables or pizza with vegetables (without cheese). The classic cake or bread and jam, are examples of combination to avoid: combine cereals or starches with sugars, gives rise to a wrong combination, since it generates fermentation.

As we have already written, but we repeat it because of absolute importance, the fruit should be consumed absolutely away from meals or half an hour before, should not be mixed even with nuts or dried fruit; nuts can be consumed at the end of a meal or as an additional ingredient in a nice mixed salad. The dried fruit can be combined well with nuts, for example: dried figs with almonds or dates with walnuts.

The next step is essential and should be done as soon as possible: remove all products of animal origin, all meat quality, including salami and all varieties of fish, eliminate from the diet milk, yogurt, cheese, butter and eggs. Legumes such as lentils, chickpeas, peas, broad beans and all types of beans can be an excellent substitute for animal products; the important thing is to make sure that these foods are fresh or dry but they should not be canned or frozen.

Reduce as much as possible the consumption of refined cereals such as pasta, white bread, white rice, pizza, superfine flour, focaccia, biscuits, rusks, croissants and all the baked goods, because these products are the ones that create absolutely more addiction. Replace refined cereals with whole grains. Valid and tasty choices can be Kamut, spelled, whole barley, red rice, black rice, brown rice, corn, millet and oats. Excellent alternatives to grain consumption may be quinoa, amaranth and buckwheat.

As you have already read, the salt, because of its deleterious characteristics, should be avoided, replace it with whole salt can be a way to limit its negative effects, but you must try to reduce its use until it is completely eliminated.

Eliminating salt from the diet is not as difficult as it seems because, even after only a week of unsalted food, the palate is refined and, in addition to no longer feeling the need to salt the food, the perceived flavors will increase in intensity, thus enhancing the true taste of food.

Increasing the intake of raw vegetables instead, is essential because it provides the right amount of fiber, minerals and enzymes that are lost in cooked foods; the ideal would be to start a meal with a salad or better with a generous mixed salad enriched with sunflower seeds, pumpkin seeds, pine nuts and avocado, seasoned with a little extra virgin olive oil cold pressed and, as an alternative to the classic vinegar, if you really can not do without it, it is recommended the use apple or lemon vinegar.

Starting the meals with vegetables will also have another positive effect: the greater sense of satiety, which raw vegetables cause, will reduce the desire to eat more, so more raw vegetables will be taken, the less harmful foods will be eaten.

The cooked vegetables instead, are excellent cooked in a pan with a little oil, better still sauté in a "wok" pot and use as a side dish or as a seasoning for all dishes; excellent and healthier if steamed or in the pressure cooker, while grilling, being too violent, releases dangerous toxins.

In place of boiled or steamed potatoes, it is better to eat well-baked potatoes; in this way the risk is reduced that their sticky starch can remain in the intestine, creating imbalances; cooking the potatoes with their peel, will make them more tasty and with an excellent supply of fiber, while the fried potatoes, due to the carcinogenic products that releases the oil heated at high temperatures, are absolutely to be avoided.

To compensate for the desire for sweets, a good alternative is to eat dried fruit (possibly organic without sugars and preservatives), which can be enjoyed freely as it nourishes without getting fat.

In the transition are also good fruit compotes instead of jams, hazelnut cream instead of Nutella (it contains too much refined sugar) and pure cocoa found in organic stores.

To quench one's thirst, the best thing is to drink centrifuged juices of fruit or vegetables, or in the absence of these pure and low-residual water, remembering to drink before or away from meals and never at the same time or immediately thereafter; therefore drinking a lot of water away from meals helps to speed up the process of elimination of waste; drinking while eating is instead a bad habit, because the liquids taken during the meal dilute the gastric juices slowing the digestion.

In bookstores you will find hundreds of books on sale offering vegan recipes, that is to say without the use of animal products; many recipes on the same topic can also be found on many online sites, just type through any search engine "vegan recipes".

A new world of tastes and flavors will become part of your diet; you will discover that the large number of dishes proposed will be excellent for eating in a healthy and natural way, without making you regret your past and unhealthy eating habits.

This first phase of transition represents the greatest difficulty for the majority of people. There is no precise advice on the exact method with which to proceed, everyone will have to make their own transition based on their needs and feelings. One piece of advice we can give you is to take all the time you need to gradually eliminate your favorite dishes, as your body will tell you the right time to remove a certain food. Being happy to eliminate some food reveals that the right time has come to proceed.

This step will lead you to the biggest change in your life; eliminating the wrong foods will allow you to discover the extraordinary positive effects that will result, your body will give you so wonderful transformations, that will never cease to amaze you.

Also just during this first phase, have been reported worldwide cases of healing of various diseases, tumors were significantly reduced and in some circumstances completely dissolved, these are just a few examples to give an idea of the potential that proper nutrition offers.

You will discover that getting rid of products of animal origin will be the simplest thing, while giving up bread, pasta, pizza and flour in general, will be for the majority of individuals quite difficult: like drugs, even refined wheat derivatives create addiction and detoxify from them it will not be an easy task.

In order not to be victims of this addiction, we advise you to replace as soon as possible all those foods produced with refined wheat flour, with as many foods produced with whole-grain cereal flour, absolutely non-GMO. During the transition phase you can be struck by a deep desire for the wrong foods, since a so total change of nutrition will have immediate effects on the neurotransmitters, while the cell transformation, which this change will require, will be achieved in longer times: the cells in fact, before they can make their change, have to wait until the connective tissue has been cleaned up.

During a continuous intake of poisons, as in the case of toxic foods, drugs or medicines, the altered functioning of the organism will become the new balance, ie the body will learn to live with that poison to survive. If at any moment the intake of this poison is interrupted, the equilibrium in being will be upset and, in the short term, the organism will not be able to recreate a new condition of stability, since for it the poison is a necessary component, even if not healthy for the balance itself, wanting again this poison.

It will therefore take a longer period of time to allow organs and glands to restore their proper functioning. An abstinence crisis, like a mad desire for a particular food, is the way in which your body reacts in an attempt to get you to take that particular substance again.

Here is the reason why during the transition you will sometimes want your "old" foods.

If you hold on for a while and do not give in to the temptation to ingest certain toxins again, all the organs and glands will restore their proper functionality and the original balance will be recovered. Over time, the desire for bad food will disappear, replaced by a consistent feeling of well-being.

Every physiological process, within a healthy body, operates in an absolute way and the various organs work masterfully in coordination with each other, thus achieving a perfect balance as only nature can do. The path of purification therefore, will be long and during the journey it will naturally come to renounce all the foods that are harmful, coming to feed on raw fruit only.

Almost all the people of today's society are no longer able to formulate their own thoughts and are unknowingly driven by a lifestyle guided by "mass thought". "Since everyone proceeds in a certain way, it means that it must be right": unfortunately it is a concept present in every individual, which makes it difficult to accept new opinions. Most people are led to believe that their habitual diet is the most suitable for the human species, perhaps because it is considered a tradition; they have never considered and analyzed the reasons and criteria on which these food choices are based. In recent decades, some expert nutritionists have given great importance to the consumption of raw fruits and vegetables.

Despite this, however, people are convinced that the main course of every meal must necessarily be cooked food, relegating raw vegetables to a side dish or consumed only by those on a diet; the fruit is then considered a kind of dessert and consumed carelessly at the end of the meal or at best as a snack.

We have already explored the topic in which it is clear that fire as a tool for altering food is a relatively recent habit; in reality, the nutrition of the human being is born raw, in the same way that all the animal species that are not in captivity naturally feed themselves.

Cooking makes food more tender and desirable, at the same time altering its nutritional characteristics, destroying micronutrients such as vitamins, antioxidants, etc.

Cooking food leads to the destruction of enzymes, the coagulation of proteins and the upsetting of satiety sensors, causing the individual to eat more than necessary. After cooking, therefore, food is no longer the food that should nourish, but rather, turns into poison and damages the whole organism. If to become edible a "food" must be cooked, it means that it is not suitable. It is therefore not a suitable food for humans.

The time has come, therefore, to stop cooking vegetables, cereals and legumes, while to compensate for the lack of carbohydrates, given by the cooked cereals, it is essential to increase considerably the quantity of fruit.

To make this nutritional leap it is necessary to have good will and considerable perseverance especially at the beginning, but it is likely that during the first steps towards a raw diet, you will naturally feel the desire to increase the consumption of raw food.

No one imagines how much time and workload the body has to sustain to restore the damage caused by cooked food; initially it will be necessary and obligatory to eat often and, given the diminution of contentment that instead produce cooked food, you will be brought to feed more abundantly.

Another cause that induces to feed more during the first phase of a raw food nutrition, is due to the fact that at the beginning the intestinal villus are not yet able to completely absorb the nutrients, because they are still obstructed by the old residues released by the products waste of inadequate foods, so the body is not yet able to sufficiently absorb all the nutrients it needs.

Considering that, as long as the body is not adequately nourished, it will send the typical sign of hunger which will lead to more nourishment; continuing to eat raw, you will also have the positive effect of cleaning up the intestinal villus, making them able to absorb a greater quantity of nutrients, causing the body to request less and less food.

Intestinal swellings, due to a greater quantity of raw fruits and vegetables, will be signs that will occur, until the intestine is completely cleaned up.

It is in these moments that most of the symptoms produced by detoxification can be presented: tiredness, a sense of weakness, light headache, discharge of mucus from the nose, etc. will be some of the annoyances that will occur, determined by the greater dissolution of poisons, facilitated by the intake of raw vegetables; this must not worry at all and, during these events, rest will be the only valid solution. By offering your body what it needs most, through the consumption of biologically appropriate and live foods, you will notice positive changes not only physical but also mental. Poisons and toxins accumulated in years of bad habits will be eliminated from your body and at the same time also various pains and discomfort will disappear. In the second phase, 100% of your diet will consist of live and nutritious foods: you will need to eat mostly from 40% to 60% with fresh fruit, from 20% to 40% with green leafy vegetables, sprouts and vegetables (peppers, tomatoes, aubergines, courgettes, pumpkin and cucumber), from 5% to 10% with avocado, olive oil, nuts, seeds and dried fruit, while condiments such as salt and vinegar, if you really can not give up immediately, will be used the least possible. Remember that even in this phase there are rules to be respected: eat fruit away from vegetables, do not mix fresh fruit with nuts, do not mix fresh fruit with dried fruit.

The fresh fruit melts the mucus that is present in the intestine forming gas: it will be normal during the first times to feel swollen, so it is always very important to eat fruit away from meals or half an hour before, even in a raw food nutrition.

Consume abundant fruit extracts at breakfast, make a mid-day meal of sweet fruit and a dinner with vegetables, avocados, seeds and chopped walnuts, represents at this stage the most suitable way to feed in the space of a day.

To take the definitive step towards the true natural nutrition of man, it is also advisable to dedicate whole days to eating only fresh fruit.

Raw foods, if prepared with dedication and competence, will be even tastier; also in this case you can find in book stores and on-line hundreds of texts that offer raw and tasty recipes, not having to give up the pleasures of the table. Switching from a raw food to an exclusively frugivorous nutrition may take a few months or a few years, depending only on you and on the degree of cleanliness that your body has reached.

This incredible food journey will gradually take you to the fabulous world of fruit.

7 ALLEGED NUTRITIONAL DEFICIENCIES

Generally, when people discover that I eat only fruit, at first they have a reaction of disbelief, then of curiosity and finally of concern. The first question that they ask is always the same: "How does it work with proteins?". Apart from serious nutrition professionals, almost all of them, out of ignorance or misinformation, believe that eating only fruit can trigger nutritional deficiencies of various kinds, not just proteins.

We must confess that I, too, before embarking on this path, like everyone else, had my own false certainties and firmly believed in the false myths that are still spread today by TV nutritional "experts" all over the world. It is for this reason that my research took place: just to understand if a fruitarian diet could cause any health problems resulting from alleged nutritional deficiencies.

After more than four years of study, assisted by personal experiences, both my and many other fruitarians, I have concluded that not only the natural diet I carry forward is without any shortage, but I have understood that it is precisely the other food styles that induced *nutritional deficiencies*. The enormous protein, vitamin, lipid, water, mineral, etc., needs, which we thought we needed, are true only following all the other diets.

INDUCED NUTRITIONAL NEEDS

Minimum quantity and maximum quality, this is the secret of perfect nutrition.

Only by following the natural diet it is possible to obtain the right nutritional needs which, as we shall see, will be minimal. The human organism is able to express maximum efficiency with the minimum structural energy, for this reason, in an efficient and clean body, the need for every single nutritive principle is extremely small. It is for this reason that a balanced diet based on fruit (for fruit I mean the types of fruit suitable for humans, as previously illustrated in the chapter on fruit), cannot under any circumstances cause nutritional deficiencies of any kind.

Only when we eat exclusively with food suitable for our species, the organism is able to achieve an almost complete organic stability.

This is the only way to trigger those physiological processes that are essential for obtaining maximum molecular efficiency. Only through this diet the molecular consumption level of each cell will be practically nil, thus reducing almost completely the daily nutritional requirements.

With the natural diet that, you get enormous benefits even immediate, not only on the physical but also on the psychic level. Neuronal cells, like all the other cells of our body, need a glucose metabolism exclusively based on fructose to work perfectly. In fact, thanks to the detoxification and the right amount of fructose that only fruit can donate, the brain cells will soon be able to bring out a great feeling of joy, contentment and serenity.

At this point in the book you will have already understood all the negative aspects that a wrong diet can cause. Now let's clarify how the induced nutritional needs are triggered.

When we eat unsuitable "food" then all the junk foods, the various animal products and their derivatives, but also legumes, cereals, oilseeds, vegetables and types of fruit unsuitable for man, a destructive process is immediately triggered, which affects every single molecule of the whole organism and this induces the demand for nutrients.

At this point, the induced nutritional needs are triggered, which are divided into induced protein requirements, induced fat and caloric requirements, induced vitamin requirements, induced mineral requirements and induced water requirements. In reality the induced requirements are much more numerous, but we believe that analyzing the most important ones is more than enough to have a comprehensive overview.

Induced protein requirement

The first induced requirement that we take into consideration is the protein one, considered the most important.

As you know by now, our blood to perform its vital functions optimally must maintain the pH value at 7.41; and as already mentioned, the only food that has this pH value, apart from the sea where life was born four billion years ago, is the apple, and more specifically the Stark red apple. The rest of the sweet fruit (apart from the acid fruit I have already discussed) has a slightly lower pH value (acid), while the fruit and fat fruits have a slightly higher (basic) value. All other foods are dangerously acidic or too basic like vegetables; all that is not fruit therefore, dangerously changes the pH of our blood causing acidity or basicity, both phenomena which, as we have seen, are very dangerous for the whole organism.

Do not think you can solve the problem by eating a salad and then consume meat, cheese and salami (very acidifying), as each food has its digestion, absorption and assimilation different times. In doing so, you will only get a period of acidosis, interspersed with a period of alkalosis, causing different damage and at different times. Keep in mind, however, that 90% of the normally consumed foods have an acidifying metabolic residue. Even basic foods contain a number of toxic and oxidizing elements that corrode us internally, subtracting electrons from all our most hidden internal structures; in short, even foods considered basic (excluding fat fruit), actually cause us a substantial acidosis.

In practice, when you are going around carelessly, probably thinking of something else, your blood goes in alarm and, to avoid letting you die, it has to put in place a series of very complex procedures and, in energetic terms, very expensive. To stay in the "range" of a vital pH, the blood is forced to remove alkaline substances from the organs, but to do this it takes time, so while the blood runs for cover, the acidifying foods just tasted literally slaughter the body.

Let us not forget that the organs, deprived of the basic elements - essential for them too - will be increasingly weakened, eventually coming to manifest those that are defined *diseases*.

Although somewhat rare, alkalosis also has the same disadvantages as acidosis.

We have reached the point where proteins come into play: at the molecular level, the biochemical action of corrosion produced by acids is devastating. Large and complex macromolecules such as proteins are those that suffer most when placed in an acidic environment; one of the first effects of an acidifying diet is to destroy an enormous quantity of proteins present in our organism: acids liberate ions $H_3 O^+$ (*Hydronium*), which, being electrically positive, because it lacks an electron, they search everywhere by finding it easily right in the "big amino acid chains".

The proteins inside our body will be so literally corroded by acids, a real subtraction of electrons, which disrupts the structure of these large molecules: this leads to the loss of their functionality, followed by total decay. This chain of events creates a pathological situation that forces the body to "desperately ask" other proteins.

In fact, tens of billions of proteins are destroyed every day because of the "standard" diet.

A vicious circle is created, induced by the feeding of high-protein and acidifying foods; the more proteins we take, the more we destroy them. This is why fruit and especially apples, possessing a pH equal or very similar to our blood, do not create all the imbalances that lead to protein deficiency. It must be made clear that proteins are not only found in animal products, but in all foods, being an integral part of the structure of every form of life.

The difference is that in fruit the concentration of protein is minimal and it is precisely this reduced concentration that makes it unable to acidify our body. Here is also explained why the acid fruit, if consumed in large quantities by those who feed only on fruit, could cause protein problems, because it is too acidifying.

While making a clear distinction between omnivorous and vegetarian, vegan or even better raw food eaters, I must stress that, due to the large quantities of foods consumed such as legumes, cereals, oilseeds, nuts, the danger of triggering the process of induced protein requirements will still be present.

Only the natural diet is free from provoking induced protein requirements. Know that the protein requirement does not depend on gender, work performed or age, but it is closely related to the type of diet.

For this reason, all the data present in the official tables regarding the presumed daily protein needs are to be considered relative and must be in fact related to the type of diet followed; a fruitarian in good health will hardly need to take more than 4 or 5 grams of protein a day, and certainly not the recommended 20 or 30 gr for all.

The mechanism that causes the remaining induced requirements is always the same, so I will avoid repeating it in the following paragraphs.

Induced lipid requirement

The unsaturated fats are the most important lipids and among these we often mention the Omega-3 and, as I will see in the dedicated chapter, they are often associated with fish or alternatively the so-called dried fruit and seeds.

However, only fruit and, in this case, more specifically the apple, contains Omega-3 of quality and immediate bioavailability. It does not matter how much of it is contained because what matters is the fact that the fruit is rich in vitamins and minerals that create the right condition for the perfect absorption and use of the lipids it contains.

Both the fish (more negative effects), the seeds, and the nuts, trigger in our body a strong acidification of the blood with all the consequences previously exposed. This triggers an induced lipid requirement; also the lipid requirement therefore, is practically nil if you follow the natural diet.

Induced glucose and caloric requirement

In addition to the previously explained mechanisms relating to acidification, with all the known consequences, with regard to the induced carbohydrate and caloric needs, I can add some considerations.

The latter is linked to an energy waste, even more relevant than the previous ones.

Precisely because of the high amount of wrong food consumed every day induces an enormous energy consumption only to digest, absorb, assimilate and above all to try to eliminate from every single cell, tissue and organ, all the toxins and poisons introduced with the nutrition itself.

It is often said that daily calories should be around 2000 Kcal per day, but this refers to those who follow an omnivorous, vegetarian, vegan or even raw food diet; in fact - apart from the natural diet - all the other food models present, more or less, big disadvantages in terms of energy expenditure.

When we eat something that is not fruit, we force the whole organism, starting from every single cell, to carry out a series of extremely heavy chemical reactions; think that, of the 2000 calories taken through the carbs, about 1600 are used only to digest, assimilate and dispose of what you eat. What a waste!

In reality, the body, to perform its normal vital functions, only needs the remaining 400 Kcal. So every day we consume more than 2,000 calories just to use 400, that's how the induced calories (glucose) requirement is born. Feeding only with fruit, thanks to the more effective metabolism of fructose, just a little more than 1000 Kcal a day are needed, which go down to 500 Kcal*, in case you eat only apples.

*Please note that this result can only be achieved gradually, only after our body has been thoroughly cleaned and accustomed to the most effective fructose metabolism. In case of particularly heavy activities, to always have an energy at the top, just increase a little more daily the amount of fruit and apples.

Induced vitamin requirement

The same argument is also valid for vitamins: if you follow the natural diet, the vitamin needs will be minimal because completely satisfied by the natural diet itself. Otherwise, following the other food regimes you can incur more or less obvious vitamin deficiencies. It is known to all for example that it is not possible to eat only animal products for a long time because the total lack of a contribution, even minimal, of fruit or vegetables, leads to the emergence of a series of diseases closely related to vitamin deficiency. An example above all, the scurvy that afflicted the long-time sailors in past centuries.

The effects described above, caused by acidifying foods, are also due to the molecular wear of vitamins; therefore, the final effect of a diet other than fruit will be the induced need for vitamins.

Also for the vitamin B12 (which I will discuss later), the same is true: any food not suitable for us increases the need for reactive catalysis of B12 both at the cytoplasmic and nucleic levels.

This entails an important molecular structural change that causes an increase of up to 170% of the B12 requirement; this is how the induced need for vitamin B12 is born, and this explains why it is never lacking in fruitarians who follow the natural diet.

Induced mineral requirement

It is always for the aforementioned reasons, due to acidifying foods, that metabolic biochemical reactions are triggered, both in the aqueous endocellular and exocellular solution: reactions which, by modifying the solvent complex, increase the requirement of oligomineral compounds very strongly.

Hence the birth of the induced needs of minerals, including iron, phosphorus, calcium and potassium. Therefore, only a natural fruit-based diet is immune to triggering physiological reactions that lead to induced mineral requirements. In short, by eating only fruit, problems of mineral deficiencies of any kind cannot occur.

Induced water requirement

Anyone will have heard that (for a whole series of reasons) you should drink at least two liters of water a day; this advice can be valid, but only for those who follow an omnivorous, vegetarian, vegan or raw food diets.

With the natural diet there is absolutely no need to drink anything, as the fruit contains about 90% of water. Indeed, calling it water is reductive, since it is a physiological liquid composed of water molecules, solvent from organic solutes contained in fruit, therefore the only true "water" suitable for our body.

As already explained in the chapter concerning water and organic minerals, the mineral waters that are normally consumed are composed of molecules solved by inorganic solutes, therefore not suitable for us. Any water not deriving from fruit (or vegetables) is a set of toxic chemicals for us, which creates a strong alteration of the organic mineral balance.

Not only that, any type of water not deriving from the plant world, being inorganic, is also acidifying precisely at the blood level. Therefore any food model different from the natural one, as well as to intoxicate us directly through the intake of acidifying foods, induces us to drink, through the stimulation of thirst, a lot of water (when it goes well, because when it goes wrong you drink wine, beer, carbonated drinks, etc.) which, as we have seen, is also harmful.

This explains how the induced water requirement is triggered, a need that can only be avoided by feeding on fresh fruit.

8 PROTEINS

In 1839 the Dutch chemist Gerhard Mulder discovered a complex organic compound, which turned out to be the main constituent of animal and plant cells.

Given the importance of this new class of molecules, the distinguished scholar decided to give them a name that well represented the primary role of all nutritious substances: "proteins" from the Greek *proteios*, that mean "of primary importance".

Proteins are chains of amino acids and the latter are rather simple organic nitrogenous compounds of different qualities and shapes, in total from fifteen to twenty types, depending on how they are counted. The chains are made up of hundreds and thousands of amino acids, which behave just like Lego bricks.

I believe, without fear to be denied, that most of us spent a few hours of childhood playing with buildings. Let's imagine taking an almost infinite number of bricks, but limiting ourselves to twenty different forms. With them we could build everything from a building to a country house, from a car to a plane, all that our imagination can imagine. This is also true for proteins. The combinations are almost endless, like the shapes they can take. Proteins are fundamental for our body, they act as enzymes, hormones, structural tissue (see skeletal muscle tissue) and transport molecules. The proteins of our organism degrade over time and must progressively be replaced.

This can happen with the ingestion of protein-based foods. What many do not know is that ingested proteins are not assimilated by the organism as such, but in the digestive system they are broken down into the constituent amino acids, which then manage to overcome the intestinal barrier and to be absorbed.

Only at this point, amino acids are used by our body to build new protein chains to replace the deteriorated ones. In practice, it is as if we had a little house built of colored Lego, we took it apart in its bricks and then, with the same ones, we built the model of an airplane. Protein-based foods contain amino acids in different percentages.

If we return to our example of bricks, we must imagine a situation in which the house is composed of all the bricks except the yellow ones; if our organism really needs those, the protein synthesis machine stops and waits for the bricks it needs. At this point, it is easy to understand why a balanced diet is important, in order to guarantee the organism the right amount of every amino acid.

This is an important condition, but not an absolute condition, because our body is able to synthesize part, if not all, of the necessary amino acids.

We finally reached the Gordian knot of the discourse: studies carried out during the last century on white rats led to the conclusion that eight amino acids, called essential, could not be synthesized by our organism. They had to be necessarily taken through the diet. If the nutritional proteins we eat have a lack of essential amino acids, the synthesis mechanism slows or stops altogether. At this point, the concept of protein quality was introduced. In other words, a scale was constructed whereby food proteins were ordered according to their quality, that is, based on their ability to supply the body with most of the essential amino acids. At the top of the Top Ten we find human flesh! That is with the perfect amino acid content we need.

The moral and health implications are evident (see *"Creutzfeldt-Jakob disease"*) which make this an impractical option. In this hypothetical ranking we find the meat of animal origin in second position. It is impossible to deny that within it all the amino acids necessary for us are present in various concentrations.

This is how, in a rather recent past, the concept of high quality protein was born, that is, it is able to completely satisfy our need for amino acids for the growth, development and maintenance of us and our children. From this classification, inevitably, the concept of low quality protein is also born, because it is poor, if not completely devoid of essential amino acids.

In a logical continuation, from all this we get the idea, deeply rooted in public opinion, that a strict vegetarian diet, vegan or the natural diet that we propose, can lead to serious protein deficiencies, with harmful consequences on the body of the crazy fools who believe in it (including the undersigned).

But let's take a step back. The situation described so far has been generated by a misunderstanding or, to be more specific, by the misplaced trust of some scholars in the research carried out, through the use of animals.

In particular, the use of laboratory mice as surrogates to humans for the study of the functioning of its metabolism. Now, it is undeniable that, as mammals like us, mice have a good deal of metabolic reactions in common with humans and their study has certainly contributed to making little light on them.

On the other hand, there are also evident differences that lead us to think that, although the basic reactions are the same, many balances and chemical mechanisms are profoundly different.

Just think, to give an example, to the case of the drug Thalidomide. Put on the market in the 60s of last century, based on studies conducted on mice, for which it turned out to be absolutely harmless, the sedative, given to pregnant women, was withdrawn from the market because cause of at least ten thousand cases of neo-natal phocomomelia, a congenital malformation of the skeleton, characterized by the lack of development of one or more limbs. A criminal lightness, to say the least. Another example, certainly less dramatic, but perhaps more relevant, refers to the protein percentages in breast milk.

The mouse pup needs for its complete development of a milk containing 9.5% of proteins, while the mother's milk has a protein content around 1%, ten times less. If we consider that the mother's milk is the main food of man, of primary and absolute importance for the complete development and growth of the newborn, we cannot help but notice how the evident diversity of composition, respect besides that of mice, like all other animals, after all, it shows a different protein requirement, a different metabolism and, ultimately, a different diet.

At this point I can state that, according to studies carried out in the middle of the last century, with good probability, eight amino acids are essential... yes, <u>but only for white mice</u>. In fact, from these studies, nothing can be said about amino acids in humans.

It is a long journey that from their discovery in 1839 brought the proteins always in greater quantities in our dishes, a road where unfortunately the breeders, the traders of cattle, the producers of salami, the industries of drugs for animal husbandry, the butchers chains, the fishing industry, slaughterhouses, hunters and related hunting-weapon industries, the freezing industry of meat and fish products, economic powers, politics and lobbies, once the deal has been discovered, with their interests have grabbed the chance; all this, in short, has contributed to paving the way for false myths, fake research, thanks to the complicity of researchers and doctors from the work not really clear and honest, of ideas that over time have to be groundless, if not dangerous for the health of man.

The mass media in this have great fault. Every day they target information based on an absolutely unfounded concept: proteins = meat. How many of us believed in it? I believed in it, my friends believed in it, my mother believed in it and my father believed in it. How many still believe in it?

Today, the truth is slowly finding its way to our consciences and our dishes. Modern and serious research, no longer based on false assumptions, are showing that the essential amino acids in humans are ultimately only two, threonine and lysine, and that from these our body can easily synthesize all the others it needs.

The good news is that these two amino acids are found in large concentrations in oily fruits, seeds, cereals, sprouts, mushrooms, spinach, asparagus and artichokes. They are present, even if in lower concentration, in almost all the fruit. As usual, Mother Nature is generous and does not spare her children anything.

As we know for over 200 years, protein chains are the main constituents of all types of cells, animals and plants, fungi, bacteria and viruses, from the small raspberry up to the giant sperm whale, proteins everywhere.

We begin to become familiar with this new awareness. In the search for the perfect food for our children and ourselves, we have been pushed to believe that to grow healthy we should eat meat: large quantities of meat. Step by step along this path we are doing together, we are discovering that this is not true, that a strict vegetarian diet does not bring harmful consequences for the organism, but rather contributes to its newfound health.

Is it possible to establish the right daily protein intake through the diet? According to the USDA (US Department of Agriculture) man needs a diet that includes a quantity of about 30 grams a day of high quality protein, that is of animal origin. In recent times, around the end of the nineteenth century, the estimated measure was 300 gr. a day, but it has been gradually reduced over time, reaching today's value.

Perhaps in the next few years it will suffer a further decrease, as we realize that, with current values, the fight against obesity in the so-called civilized countries will prove to be absolutely ineffective. It is evident that the path towards the right values must proceed in stages, since the USDA is susceptible to the control of food lobbies, each step taken is the result of a struggle between interests of considerable importance. But how do you know what the right intake is?

Beyond the costly experiments carried out by scholars of half the world, the truth is that nature comes to us and provides us with an incredibly simple tool to assess how much must be the protein needs of a man: once again I talk about breast milk. Or, to be more precise, the value of protein concentration in human milk.

As we have already seen in reference to laboratory mice and as I have dealt with in much more detail in the chapter dedicated to it, it is an extremely low value 10-11gr / L. Given the small quantity of milk consumed by an infant, about 100 ml a day, during the initial phase of his life, which corresponds, however, at the time of greater growth and development (in fact he doubles its weight in a few days), we can easily understand how the daily protein requirement is actually very small. This is due to the incredible ability of man to exploit every single ingested molecule, combined with the possibility of synthesizing himself the amino acids he needs to build his body.

It is possible, at this point, to suppose that the incredible quantity of proteins of animal origin ingested during his life, could compromise the delicate metabolic balance of man, leading to the onset of diseases that undermine the quality of life itself, up to lead to premature death?

In his book "*The China Study*" Dr. T. Colin Campbell describes the results of a research on the mortality rates of twelve different types of cancer in more than 2,400 Chinese counties, with a total sample of 880 million people (96% of the population), which involved 650,000 operators on Chinese territory.

Thanks to the statistical data collected, in what has rightly been defined the most ambitious biomedical research ever undertaken by man and others, countless, collected in twenty-seven years by Dr. Campbell himself, with the help of a team of researchers formed by American and Chinese scientists, it has been possible to demonstrate incredible and unexpected correlations between the onset and development of many types of cancer, diseases affecting the circulatory system, obesity, etc. and nutrition based on proteins and animal fats.

I would like to be clear, the study enjoys the esteem of the entire scientific community worldwide, it has been conducted with the rigor and precision expected of a team of professionals and scientists with unquestionable credentials and it has resulted in thousands of articles published by major international scientific journals. The study clearly shows that a diet rich in proteins and fats of animal origin promotes the origin and development of various types of cancer, including breast, prostate, colon and liver cancer.

Furthermore, it creates an unexpected correlation between animal protein intake and high cholesterol levels in the blood, with the consequent development of hypertension, angina pectoris, heart attack and stroke. The research identifies in a protein in particular the ability to favor the establishment and progress of malignant cancers, induced by external carcinogens substances and viruses.

What does it mean? It means that by feeding on that specific protein we facilitate the birth of a cancer, for example of the liver, following the modification of the cellular DNA promoted by an external agent, as, for example, *aflatoxin*, due to fungal infection of peanuts. And yet, that protein helps cancer find the breeding ground suitable for its development and its proliferation in the human body, leading to death.

The research shows that, following the nutritional suspension of that precise protein of animal origin, there is a regression of the cancer itself, until healing; and in individuals who follow a strictly vegan diet, in the total absence of that same protein, there is almost complete immunity from the nefarious effects of the carcinogenic substance, no DNA mutation, zero cancer.

Did I manage to intrigue you? The protein of which I have described the nefarious effects in the last paragraphs is none other than casein. 87% of cow's milk proteins are made of casein. It is found in cheeses, in yoghurts, in the powdered milk we give to our children, in all dairy products and in all the products on the market that have cow's milk among the ingredients.

Unfortunately there are autoimmune diseases. The human immune system, usually very efficient, in some individuals turns its own attack towards the cells of your body. This unpleasant and serious inconvenience gives rise to very serious, painful, disabling and, in many cases, fatal diseases. The reasons that lead to the development of an auto-immune disease are many, complex and to date, not fully clarified, but, among them, it seems that feeding on animal proteins is a probable cause. Every cell in our body has certain proteins, the antigens, on its surface, called the cell membrane. These proteins are like fingerprints, different from individual to individual, allowing the immune system to always distinguish between cells belonging to your body and foreign cells, in technical jargon "*self*" and "*not-self*".

During digestion, it may happen that some ingested animal proteins are not completely separated into the constituent amino acids, but that parts of the chains of which they are formed are able to overcome the intestinal barrier and enter the blood circulatory bed. Immediately, the immune system intervenes, the protein chains are recognized as not-self and attacked. One of the most incredible mechanisms of the immune system is the creation of antibodies specific to the not-self invading antigens.

Thanks to these antibodies, following a new attack of a not-self antigen, previously recognized, the reaction of the immune system becomes fast and absolutely efficient. The point is that some of the protein chains, able to cross the intestinal barrier during digestion, have a marked resemblance to self antigens of our body.

The problem finally takes shape. Normally, the immune system is equipped with complicated *feedback* mechanisms that allow it to easily recognize not-self antigens from self antigens, even if apparently identical, and then proceed to a selective attack. For reasons not yet clarified, these security systems in certain individuals, and fortunately rarely, fail. Then the unimaginable happens.

The immune system no longer distinguishes between self and not-self similar antigens. Antibodies are created and launched in a blind attack that does not distinguish the friend from the enemy, in a tremendous reaction and, ultimately, self-destructive.

This is the case of a well-known autoimmune disease that affects millions of people every year in all nations and at all social levels, *type 1 diabetes*. Casein seems to be, once again, the cause of a terrible disease. This protein, in its amino chain, has accentuated similarities with the antigens that coat the cells of the islands of Langerhans, organelles present in the Pancreas, for the synthesis and release in the blood bed of the hormones insulin and glucagon, in order to control the concentration of the glucose in the blood. In the aforementioned people, the presence of parts of the casein protein chain in the blood triggers the blind antibody reaction, which also attacks the cells of the Langerhans islands, destroying the ability of our body to produce the two hormones.

The thing happens step by step, but in the long run it has death as its sole result. Hence the need for diabetes patients to continue insulin injections in order to lead a life that is at least apparently normal. Once again, I wonder how much milk should flow in white rivers, before one realizes its danger.

Far from having even just touched on the complete and exhaustive treatment of proteins, I stop at these few examples, postponing the reader to much more exhaustive publications. At this point, I would like to dwell for a moment on the criticism of mass medicine, for those who have decided to abandon food of animal origin in favor of a strict vegan diet.

It will then be true that they are crazy? Meanwhile, the most obvious benefit: no milk and dairy products, no casein. Just for this, life expectancy takes a decisive leap forward. Then, no animal proteins around, like self antigens, to do damage to our body. The consequences on auto-immune diseases are therefore evident. And again, no fertiliser to enrich the growth of tumors and cancers, many toxic mutagens substances of DNA, see aflatoxin, become harmless... on this subject Dr. Campbell has much to say.

The proteins of plant origin supply all the amino acids we need and, on the other hand, if this were not so, where would the herbivores or the frugivore species take them? And with these, do not think only of the cattle, but the gorillas, our very close cousins and, I would say rather healthy for supposed amino deficiencies. Still the animals, you'll say.

True. But far more similar to us than a laboratory mice, I will answer.

Essential amino acids? Speech passed, our body finds all the amino acids it needs in the nature that surrounds it, just stretch a hand and pick a beautiful fruit. Even if all were not present, we are able to recover the amino acids from the degradation of the protein chains that have terminated their life cycle in our organism and if, even so, some amino acids continue to lack, well we can synthesize them ourselves.

Daily protein requirement? I think this point is clear to everyone: the daily requirement must necessarily be minimal. We get that from latest medical research, breast milk tells it us too and from the low percentage of protein in fruit, coincidentally, the two percentages are perfectly identical.

Still doubts? In China thirty years ago, the percentage of colon cancer in the population, with a poor and almost exclusively vegetarian diet, was 0, *zero*. Today, with the advance of the western diet, rich in proteins of animal origin, that same percentage has become the same as USA !

That the evil of kings, as it was called in the Middle Ages, for obvious reasons, cancer, must find its causes in food?

All of the above is just the tip of the iceberg on top of which our health wobbles in a balance that is unstable, to say the least. The very serious consequences for it, linked to an excessive diet based on proteins of animal origin, every day acquire more and more remarkable scientific and medical evidence.

In a world in which the fight against cancer, which takes away our loved ones, if it does not directly affect ourselves, it is being lost by official medicine at the very high cost of money, but still higher in human lives. Of all this, public opinion must be informed, to give each of us the opportunity to choose and the opportunity to live a better life in a friendly, strong and healthy body.

Finally, more importantly, to give us the opportunity to guarantee our children the greatest good: the quality of a joyful life in this so beautiful and unique world. Before

closing the speech let me say a few words of optimism. The research shows this, even for us who have lived in the dark of this information there is a great hope of improving our health, losing weight, solving the endless problems and ailments that haunt us every day. Abandoning the omnivorous diet, embracing a strict vegan diet and by strict I mean without milk and derivatives, eggs or fish; finally, eating large quantities of fruit, no magic, no miracles, only certainties.
Your life can change for the better.

9 VITAMINS

Vitamin, the *anime of life*, from the German term Vitamin. This was the name coined by the researcher Casimir Funk, in 1912, after identifying an amine group in the thiamine structure, isolated the year before.

Later, around the Thirties of the century, Elmer Verner McCollum, managed to separate from milk what he called a *fat-soluble factor A* and *water-soluble factor B*. Two substances, until then unknown, indispensable for the growth of laboratory animals. These were the steps that gave rise to the discovery of a new class of substances essential to life, *vitamins* precisely.

Vitamins are essential elements, our body cannot synthesise them alone, but must be ingested with the diet. Exceptions are *vitamin D*, synthesized from cholesterol through sunlight exposure to parts of the body, and *niacin*, synthesized from tryptophan, an essential amino acid.

That of vitamins are not a group of chemically homogeneous substances. In fact, they differ both in the structure and at the level of biological action mechanisms. Furthermore, the concentrations necessary for their effectiveness, as well as those present in foods, are very low, at the milligram and microgram levels. These are the factors that have made the discovery so difficult and late. Initially, the nomenclature of vitamins was followed according to the order with which they were isolated, A, B, C, D and so on. Today we prefer to assign names based on function, so we observe that vitamin K derives its ending from the Danish Koagulation, coagulation, being a fundamental substance for its control.

To give an order to this class of substances, it was decided to divide them into two subclasses: *water-soluble vitamins* and *fat-soluble vitamins*. Two characteristics that explain its behavior and allow us to understand its functioning mechanisms more easily.

The water-soluble vitamins (*thiamin, riboflavin, niacin, vitamin B6, folacin, vitamin B12, ascorbic acid (C), biotin and pantothenic acid*) are generally absorbed rapidly by the walls of the digestive system and the solubility in the blood allows easy transport in all the organism. These substances are not accumulated in the tissues, the excess concentrations are quickly eliminated at the level of the kidneys.

Because of their inability to be stored, the water-soluble vitamins should be taken regularly with the diet, so as not to start deficiency phenomena that can lead to diseases such as *scurvy* (vitamin C deficiency) or *pellagra* (vitamin D deficiency). The excess intake of these vitamins does not normally have contraindications, if not kidney fatigue with, in case of abuse, possible formation of stones.

Most of the water-soluble vitamins function as *coenzyme*, without them the enzymes that regulate the main functions of the life of all living beings, not only of man therefore, cannot proceed.

The physical and chemical characteristics of water-soluble vitamins make them very delicate.

The fat-soluble vitamins (*A, D, E, K*), are absorbed at the intestinal level in the same way as lipids and, like these, they can be stored, especially by the liver. Their elimination, in case of excess, is slow and difficult, this can lead to a real poisoning of the organism. Fat-soluble vitamins intervene in all the typical mechanisms of superior animals, such as tissue growth and differentiation, fluidity and mineral blood homeostasis, etc.

This group of such heterogeneous substances participates in every aspect of the life of living organisms. It is essential to understand its importance. The deficiency of any vitamin leads to disastrous consequences for the body; pellagra, scurvy, beri-beri, are only the most known diseases, but there are others more subtle, such as: fatigue, irritability, sleep and memory disorders, lack of appetite, constipation; stomatitis of the oral mucosa, seborrhea; problems in energy metabolism and breathing; dermatitis, eczema and problems with the structural and functional integrity of the nervous system; breakdown of collagen in connective tissues; problems with blood coagulation; danger of deformation of the fetus during pregnancy; damage in the regulation of gene expression of proteins of crucial importance in cell metabolism; inability to regulate calcium homeostasis, osteoporosis; hemolytic anemia; effects on the control and elimination of free radicals, cancer risk; and yet so many diseases that it would take a book to describe them all.

Fortunately, however, the diet of modern man makes virtually impossible any kind of vitamin deficiency, unless there is an aberrant dietary behavior or a particularly dramatic situation, see the wars affecting the poorest African countries, where the lack of choice in food, if not the complete lack of it, leads to the consequent hypovitaminosis.

In addition there could be deficiencies related to poor food storage or improper preparation. In fact, the vitamins are rather delicate, easily meeting oxidation and rancidity. Water-soluble vitamins, for example, tend to be dispersed in cooking liquids and disintegrate due to the heat itself. The deficiency may also be due to other factors, such as diseases at the gastro-intestinal level, which slow down or block absorption. A pernicious anemia is a typical example, sometimes caused not by the lack of vitamin B12 intake in the diet, but rather by the lack of a protein, secreted by the gastric mucosa, necessary for the absorption of the vitamin itself. In cases of this kind we talk about secondary deficiencies, to distinguish them from those related to the diet.

On the contrary, a problem that may arise in our day is the excessive intake of vitamins. As we have seen, if it is a matter of water-soluble vitamins, it is quickly resolved by the kidneys, but this should not lead us to underestimate the problem.

A prolonged *excess*, in fact, has bad influences on the elimination mechanisms, with all that entails, as we have underlined several times in this book. Concerning the class of fat-soluble vitamins, excess leads to rather serious, even irreversible pathologies. To better understand the problem, I will make a small reference to vitamin A. It is fundamental, since it comes into play in many important mechanisms: it acts in the mediation of gene expression; acts at the retina level; it acts in the differentiation of the epithelial cells and in the morphological and functional maintenance of mucous membranes such as conjunctival and those of the respiratory tract, gastrointestinal and urogenital; then, again, of embryogenesis, in growth and reproduction, etc.

The striking thing is that, despite all these functions, the daily requirement of this vitamin is about 600/700 µg, respectively for women and men, very minimal. This makes us understand how easy it is to overcome this dose with the nutrition of western countries, based on meat and milk derivatives. Why? Soon said.

The vitamin A complex is made up of two groups of substances, the actual vitamin A present in food of animal origin, and the carotenoids present in food of plant origin. The first group, is nothing but vitamin A synthesized by animals during their life from *carotenoids*, ingested in turn, and accumulated in their meat. The second, instead, is a group of pigments, generally orange, some of which, called *pro-vitamin A*. They are used, at the level of our gastric mucosa, for the synthesis of new vitamin A. The most important of these is *B-carotene*.

Carotenoids have many other functions in our body, as well as being precursors of vitamin A.

For example, they are magnificent anti-oxidants, fundamental for eliminating free radicals, guilty of diseases such as cancer. The diet too rich in meat and animal products, leads to a high intake of vitamin A of animal origin, with an excessive accumulation that, in the long run, can lead to poisoning, let alone then, if we add a nice dose of vitamin supplements!

This cannot happen in a vegetarian diet, since an excess of carotenoids does not involve the equivalent excess of vitamin A, not being completely transformed into this substance, but only in the part that the body needs. In addition there are no contraindications in case of excess of the latter.

The vegetarian diet based on fruit and absolutely fresh products allows the right amount of vitamin, always avoiding the risk of deficiencies, but also and above all of vitamin excess. Below is a list for information of the vitamins discovered to date.

Vitamin A: Retinoids (and Carotenoids as provitamin A)

Vitamins B: initially reputed single vitamin then proved to be a group of water-soluble vitamin (B)

Vitamin C: Ascorbic acid, the most common and powerful antioxidant

Vitamin D: initially reputed single vitamin then proved to be a group of liposoluble pro-hormones (D)

Vitamin E: Liposoluble antioxidant tocopherols

Vitamin F: Essential fatty acids (Omega-3 and Omega-6)

Vitamin G: Riboflavin or Vitamin B2 (belonging to Group B)

Vitamin H: Biotin or Vitamin B8 (belonging to Group B)

Vitamin I: Inositol or Vitamin B7 (belonging to Group B)

Vitamin J: Choline, an essential nutrient sometimes combined with Group B

Vitamin K: Complex group of compounds (K from the German Koagulation, Coagulation)

Vitamin L: Anthranilic acid (a metabolite of Tryptophan)

Vitamin M: Folic acid or Vitamin B9 or Vitamin Bc (belonging to Group B)

Vitamin N: Alpha Lipoic Acid - ALA (or thioctic acid), a powerful antioxidant both liposoluble and water-soluble

Vitamin P: Bio-flavonoids. Powerful water-soluble antioxidants (Vitamin C adjuvants)

Vitamin PP: Niacin or Vitamin B3 (belonging to Group B) acronym of English Pellagra Preventive

Vitamin Q: Ubiquinone or Coenzyme Q-10 (CoQ10)

Vitamin R: abbreviated para aminobenzoic acid PABA, or Vitamin B10 (belonging to Group B)

Vitamin S: Pteroyl-hepta glutamic acid or Vitamin B11 (belonging to Group B)

Vitamin T: Tocotrienols, food factor of Sesame seeds (belonging to Vitamin E)

Vitamin U: Methylmethionine or S-methyl-L-methionine, substance present in some plants

Vitamin V: probably related to the coenzyme NAD / NADH

Vitamin W: Pantothenic acid or Vitamin B5 (belonging to Group B)

Vitamin X: currently not used

Vitamin Y: Pyridoxine or Vitamin B6 (belonging to Group B)

Vitamin Z: Zinc, essential nutrient proposed (and not accepted) as a vitamin

10 VITAMIN B12

Vitamin B12 seems to be one of the favorite subjects of omnivores, as evidence to justify their food choice. Many vegans frightened by superficial information about it, feel obliged to integrate their diet with supplements of B12. This unnecessary bogey on the B12 is also one of the reasons why many vegetarians do not want to give up eggs and dairy products, convinced that such foods are essential to take the "mythical" vitamin B12. On-line there are often articles written by "pseudo-vegetarian" experts who stress the health problems attributable to vitamin B12 deficiency, related to those who follow vegan diets.

In this chapter we will try to shed light on the topic B12, so as to clarify the ideas also to those who, while supporting a natural diet, is worried about incurring any vitamin deficiencies. Doctors who blindly follow indications from scientific organizations accredited by the World Health Organization (WHO) are sometimes inclined to hypothesize vitamin B12 deficiencies in people who follow vegetarian and especially vegan diets.

Who feeds on a vegan raw food diet or based on fruit, vegetables, nuts, seeds and sprouts, has B12 values that are usually found on 90-120 pg / ml (*picograms, ie, billionths of a gram per milliliter of blood*); even if they are absolutely correct values, they do not fit with official data and obviously this can create false alarms, urging doctors to propose absolutely useless "cures" of integration and indeed, as you will understand later, often harmful.

The doubts about the vitamin B12 deficiency are born because they take as "sacred" references the tables drawn up by official entities such as the American FDA (Food and Drug Administration), but these tables were made analyzing absurd data. The minimum level of B12 in the blood, according to these "official" tables, should be around 156 pg / ml, arbitrarily changed recently. In fact, before the 70s, another scientific entity, the WHO (World Health Organization), had rightly fixed this value at 80 pg / ml. Keep in mind that the FDA is the same entity that in the second half of the last century brought the minimum daily protein quota to 300 grams / day, modified today, after twenty years and numerous embarrassing adjustments, to say the least, at 30 grams / day (however still too high).

These tables are written analyzing the dietary habits of high-protein diets consumers, who feed on meat, milk, cheese, eggs, etc. every day. Having established that B12 is mostly found in animal products, it is obvious that, if we analyze the omnivores that feed on them every day, the B12 value is necessarily high. The expert editors of the FDA consider this value (exaggeratedly high) as the average of the population, thus considering it correct; an absurd way of working, because this datum simply represents the snapshot of a reality in which the population is nourished and very ill. I believe that a table of so important values should be drawn up observing scientific data concerning the true state of health of a healthy human being and not based on averages referring to evidently sick people, just like the Americans who, as we know, are at the top of the rankings among the peoples with the highest percentage of pathologies attributable to the SAD (*Standard American Diet*).

The FDA still keep going and, continuing to follow its modus operandi, has set also the maximum value of B12, even over 1000 pg / ml, a value of almost seven times higher than the minimum: our suspicion is that this differential was established solely to justify the busted values of meat consumers around the world.

So do not be frightened by the B12 values considered low, and do not integrate your diet with eggs and milk, thus undermining the benefits of a non-carnivorous diet. With low amounts of B12, all the values of vitamin B, including homocysteine and B9, are in equilibrium with each other, moreover with the right contribution of the other vitamins, the minimum values of B12 make the blood much more fluid, eliminating risks of stroke and heart attack.

As we mentioned with regard to the induced deficiencies, those who follow a natural frugivorous diet can not present vitamin B12 deficiencies, whereas for omnivores, vegetarians and vegans, a possible problem due to B12 deficiency is never caused by the quantity taken, which it is always more than sufficient for the needs of the organism, but rather it could be a problem deriving from incorrect assimilation, or from other factors that compromise its bioavailability.

Probably few people know that a large quantity of B12 is present in the sewers of the urban areas; this shows that the majority of people, even taking it in large quantities with carnivorous food, eliminate it almost entirely.

As for the trace elements, also vitamin B12, to be efficient, does not require to be present in large quantities, so the problem is not the dose you ingest, but the ability that your body has to assimilate it: it is obvious that, if you feed yourself with unsuitable products or with the right foods, but denatured by cooking or industrial processes, the toxins released from these foods will engorge the lymphatic and blood system, making the assimilation of vitamins, including B12, very difficult.

Who claims that B12 is present only in animal tissues and therefore unavailable in the plant world, concludes that the only acidce of supply is in meat, fish, eggs and dairy products.

But then, the cow that you eat where takes the B12?

In fact, traces of B12 are found in the plant world even if in small quantities. To counter the hypothesis, that those who do not eat animals cannot have adequate values of B12, we report a study conducted by a French scientist which shows why the people who eat only fruit and vegetables do not show deficiency of B12.

The French scientist Corentin Louis Kervran (1901-1983) was a chemist and physicist, as well as a university lecturer specialized in natural hygiene, in occupational medicine and an expert in agriculture. Kervran began his research in 1935 and only in 1961 made his theory known, but of course he was immediately opposed and ridiculed by scientists of the time. His research was then shelved and hidden, just by doctors and colleagues, but fortunately, in 1974 the CERN in Geneva, the most important nuclear research center, confirmed the theories of Kervran.

The experiment conducted by the scholar was simple and elementary and allowed him to demonstrate how it is possible to transmute potassium into calcium: the experiment involved some hens who were given a diet strictly free of calcium, although they were nevertheless able to lay eggs with shells; the fact that the hens continued to lay eggs complete with shell seemed strange, since the shell is composed mainly of calcium; the cases are two, or the hens took the calcium from their bones, or they obtained it in another way.

The sensational discovery was that the organism of the hens managed to transmute the potassium, of which their diet was rich, into calcium. Below, other scientists in addition to dr. Kervran, performed the same type of experiment on other animals and on some plants obtaining the same incredible result, the transmutation of the elements.

The ancient alchemists were always looking for a method that would help them to transmute the elements, probably they could not. The results of Kervran's experiments indicate that nature is able to perform such transmutation very easily.

The French studies showed us the transformation of potassium into calcium through a weak nuclear reaction: without release of energy, one atom generated another atom without generating or absorbing heat. The same transmutation process can be applied to vitamin B12. Let's go back for a moment to potassium and calcium. These have near numbers in the periodic table of elements, potassium has an atomic number of 19 (19 atomic particles per nucleus, neutrons and protons) and calcium has an atomic number of 20. One of the basic elements of the B12 structure is cobalt whose atomic number is 27, only one more than the atomic number of iron, 26. These chemical characteristics, or the proximity of the corresponding atomic numbers, make it possible to transmute both calcium in potassium (as in the case of eggs), and therefore cobalt in iron (as for B12). In summary, Kervran's experiments prove that it is possible to obtain cobalt (vitamin B12) from iron, demonstrating how cows, horses and herbivores in general, are able to produce B12 feeding on grass alone. It is therefore presumable that the human being is also able to obtain the right amount of B12 by consuming foods rich in iron.

Cobalt, which constitutes vitamin B12, is a heavy metal, a toxic and poisonous element. It is therefore clear that if taken in high quantities, B12 becomes toxic.

For this reason *cobalamin* (vitamin B12) is present in fruit and vegetables in low quantities that are difficult to detect; in fact, nature has established that the main food of man should contain the right and very low quantity of vitamin B12.

It is not necessary to eat animal products, to take pills or supplements to have sufficient supply of B12 coenzymes. Besides fruits and vegetables, also seeds, nuts and sprouts contain them in a form available to human beings.

Beware, the true deficiency of vitamin B12 is actually a problem for the body, but this applies to the whole complex of vitamin B, ie B1, B2, B3, B5, B6, B9 and B12, as it is shown that the group of vitamin B always works in synergy. The reasons for these deficiencies are complex and must be assessed individually, case by case, but we cannot speak of vitamin B12 deficiency isolated from the others.

As already mentioned above, the real problem in a possible deficiency is not related to the quantity ingested, but to the quantity absorbed by the organism. The reasons for which cobalamin or other vitamins are not absorbed are numerous: *celiac disease* (gluten allergy), *reductive operations of the intestines, idiopathic steatorrhea* and *presence of worms*.

One of the main causes of vitamin malabsorption is due to the presence of *gastric atrophy*. It occurs after years of feeding with wrong foods that cause chronic irritation of the gastric mucosa. If we continue to ingest harmful food, we induce continuous indigestion in the stomach, with all the various consequences.

If the body is unable to absorb the nutrients, they will only feed the bacteria; stomach and intestine will be increasingly irritated and inflamed by bacterial decomposition and gastroenteritis. Gastritis, colitis, etc., will be the consequence and when conditions worsen, mechanisms will be triggered that will lead, in addition to probable tumors or ulcers, also the aforementioned atrophy.

Like other health problems, even gastrointestinal disorders can and should be fought by removing the causes, that is to say following a diet that is able to restore the immune system to its full efficiency, thus allowing the body to heal itself. Apart from those who have already undergone surgery to the intestines, in which case the situation is more complex, all the others who have vitamin deficiencies (including B12), through a natural diet, trying to do a minimum of physical exercise and taking a bit of sun, can go back to absorb all the B12 and other necessary vitamins.

We have therefore established that by eating with foods of vegetable origin there will be no lack of B12, as there will be no lack of any other nutrient necessary for the correct development and maintenance of the body. However, it is important to underline that the organism will have to be "clean" enough, before being able to digest and completely absorb the various nutrients, including B12.

The active vitamin B12 co-enzymes are also found in the mouth bacteria, around the tonsils, between the teeth, in the nasal pharynx, at the base of the tongue and in other neighboring places. Coenzyme B12 is the form with which vitamin B12 is present in animals and plants, but these coenzymes are extremely delicate and cease to function when they are removed from their natural habitat. Sometimes, regardless of the type of diet, a supplement of B12 is prescribed by doctors through non-natural supplements, but these almost never lead to positive effects, since all vitamin B12 supplements contain cyanocobalamin, a substance that the body is not able to use.

The confusion on this subject comes from the fact that often biochemists, doctors and various authors, use the term B12 referring however to *cyanocobalamin*. Cyanocobalamin is the semi-synthetic vitamin B12 which, by means of cyanide, is chemically extracted from animal tissues; B12 supplements made with this procedure, in addition to not bringing any real benefit, poison those who use it because cyanide is toxic. Cyanocobalamin, once it reaches the blood bed, dissociates into cyanide and cobalamin, the cyanide binds to potassium forming potassium cyanide which is a powerful poison. The organism, to stop this highly toxic reaction, attacks the synthetic supplement by eliminating it as quickly as possible.

This explains why about 90% of cyanocobalamin taken with supplements is eliminated within twenty-four hours and subsequently found in the sewers.

Another method for obtaining B12 is by means of an extraction procedure which takes place with the aid of columns of coal and nitrogen which, however, still results in cyanocobalamin, two different methods for obtaining the same toxic substance, completely different from that that is found in nature, but that many experts erroneously continue to call vitamin B12.

A possible lack of B12 cannot be resolved through supplements: those who take cyanocobalamin supplements show an apparent benefit, due to the production of adrenaline by the body that gives a false vitality, caused by the injection of a poisonous substance, not solving at all the problem due to the lack of vitamin. The intake of these synthetic substances does not therefore provide any type of integration and moreover, due to the effort the organism is subjected to inactivate the cyanide, there is a huge waste of energy. Excessive stimulation causes a gradual worsening of health as a whole.

Supplements, tablets or injections of B12 do not work because as it is now clear, synthetic substances act differently than natural ones. People can be made to believe that synthetic vitamins bring benefit, but it is just advertising campaigns. Only natural vitamins should be taken, including those of group B, since only natural ones have the corresponding coenzymes and all the factors of group B (including those still unknown by science).

It is always dangerous to resort to a single vitamin and not to all of its group. In this way you can run into sudden changes, deficiencies and excesses, compared to the other vitamins of the same complex. For example, vitamin B12 is essential in DNA synthesis but only in competition with folic derivatives, ie vitamin B9.

As you have already read in the chapter on induced needs, the better the diet and the lower the requirement for vitamin B12; we can therefore summarize by stating that all the controversies related to B12 are useless: if nature has predisposed a certain quantity of this vitamin on the peel of the fruit and on other vegetables, it means that the needs of a man's organism, free from slag and toxins, will be widely

satisfied, simply by following the natural diet.

To enjoy excellent health, therefore, it is useless to worry about a single vitamin, but it is only through all the vitamins, the organic minerals, the right dose of protein and all the other necessary elements that one can achieve true well-being. Life is much more than a vitamin, it is a set of complicated processes, chemical reactions, interactions and bonds, so complex procedures that science still cannot fully demonstrate.

Nourish only with raw plant foods, try not to take drugs, coffee, stimulants, sugar and smoke as sequestering agents of vitamins: only in this way you can achieve excellent health and without worrying about individual vitamin deficiencies, including B12.

11 CALCIUM, SODIUM AND POTASSI-UM

Life is linked to a whole series of mechanisms that, from the simplest to the most complex, must work perfectly and above all in perfect harmony with each other. At any moment, when one of these mechanisms, even the most insignificant, gets jammed, the whole system suffers, the marvelous machine that is the living organism suffers and the functioning is compromised.

All this is said to introduce a vast and very complex subject, which we will only cover superficially: the role of calcium, sodium, potassium and other inorganic minerals in the functioning of our organism.

This class of substances groups macro, micro and trace elements. They are all molecules that our body needs, even in really microscopic doses, but of which it is not able to handle the synthesis, that is, they must be acquired through food.

Calcium

Of calcium, I have already discussed in many parts of our little treaty.

It covers innumerable tasks in our body, the best known of which is the fundamental component of the bones. The bone tissue, in fact, has an extremely complex structure, characterized by *connective tissue*, in which the blood and lymphatic vessels pass, with the task of bringing the nutrients and removing the waste substances, and from the *nerves*, which are responsible for conveying the information necessary for bone cells. The latter constitute the living compartment, properly called the bone tissue, and are formed by *osteoblasts*, with the task of building the tissue, *osteoclasts*, which, in opposition to the former, have the task of demolishing it, *osteocytes*, which keep the first two classes alive and the tissue itself. Connective tissue and bone cells form, however, only about 30% of the bone, the remaining 70% is made up of *minerals*, in particular from *hydroxyapatite*, in turn formed by 60% of *calcium*, 30% of *phosphorus* and remaining 10% of *oxygen* and *hydrogen*. In an individual of about 70 kilos, calcium accounts for about 1.5% of the total weight, about a kilo. Osteoclasts demolish about 0.5 grams of tissue a day, so over 5/6 years it can be said that the whole mineral component of the bone tissue is completely replaced. From a structural point of view this is important, since the bones and especially the lines of force that allow the bones to discharge, for example, to the ground, the weight of the body during walking, or during the lifting of a load, are gradually changed to better adapt to the different demands imposed by the environment.

But this is not enough, in fact, calcium intervenes in the fundamental mechanism of human pH control. The continuous work of demolition and reconstruction of the bones has, therefore, the purpose of modifying the levels of blood calcium to buffer the acidity, due, as mentioned previously, to our continuous exposure to chemical and biological pathogenic agents, not least, the feeding based on highly acidifying foods of animal origin, smoking and alcohol.

Another aspect not yet taken into consideration is the role of calcium in muscle contraction. The latter, fundamental for allowing us to move and interact at all levels with the world, is the result of a series of rigidly coordinated reactions that, at the intracellular level of the muscle fibers, allow its movement.

Upon the arrival of the electrical impulse that commands the beginning of the contraction, the surface of the muscle cells is depolarised, that is, there is a variation of electric charge, which leads to the release of calcium in the form of an ion, Ca ++. This reaches the *troponin* protein and, by binding to it, causes it to change its shape, starting the chain of reactions that will result in muscle movement. Without calcium we cannot move, swallow, breathe and the heart cannot beat.

Calcium is also implicated in the processes of the *cascade blood coagulation*, in *neuronal activation*, in the *control of the secretion of hormones and growth factors*, in *gene transcription* and in many *metabolic cell activities*.

All this explains why our body is particularly careful in controlling blood and intracellular calcium levels. Due to renal and hepatic dysfunctions and diet-related problems, important concentration variations may also occur.

Hypercalcemia has symptoms such as fatigue, nausea, vomiting, constipation and thirst, gradually worsening until it leads to psychic disorders with mental confusion, delirium and coma. But that's not all, kidney problems can arise due to the formation of calcium phosphate deposits and finally severe cardiac arrhythmias. *Hypocalcemia*, on the other hand, causes alterations to the electrical potential of neuromuscular membranes, cramps and tetany, laryngeal spasms and convulsions, severe cardiac arrhythmias that can result in heart block and death.

If it is important for our body to keep the blood and intracellular calcium levels constant, it is perhaps even more important to keep the ratio between calcium and phosphorus concentrations constant, which must be between 3:1 and 2:1 (to be precise, 2.6: 1).

Phosphorus, that we will only mention, is a very important substance. It is the foundation of the cytoplasmic membranes of every living being on earth (formed precisely by phospholipids).

In the form of *ATP, adenosine triphosphate*, it is the vehicle and energy storage necessary for each metabolic reaction. Phosphorus is one of the fundamental constituents of nucleic acids, DNA and RNA. In the form of *inorganic phosphate* is the second component, by quantity, of the hydroxyapatite of the bone tissue and enters, together with calcium, in the mechanisms associated with the pH buffer control.

The rigid ratio between calcium and phosphorus is very important because it affects the release and absorption rates of the two minerals at the level of the bone tissue.

It affects the ability of the digestive system to take them and the ability of the kidney to eliminate or reabsorb them. An example for everyone: as we read in the chapter dedicated to cow's milk, the ratio between calcium and phosphate of cow's milk is 1:1. It is useless therefore to continue to assume it, convinced by the media of its goodness for our bones.

Calcium, in addition, compared to phosphorus is not absorbed by the intestine. And if absorbed, it must be immediately eliminated at the renal level, with the risk of formation of painful stones. The same end will make calcium ingested with synthetic supplements sold in pharmacies: these change the relationship between the two minerals and, far from helping us, force our body to a super-work to eliminate the excess.

Remember the nefarious effects of hypercalcemia. Although classical food science, or better, media, continues to argue that we must seamlessly integrate our calcium deposits, there is indisputable evidence that natural food, although apparently less rich in calcium, allows us to keep our mineral levels at the right values. This is due to the exact relationship between the minerals taken, as well as to its characteristic of helping to keep the organism at the right pH value.

As a consequence, the need to provide the buffer mechanisms decreases, these necessary for maintaining the balance between acids and bases, leading to an evident consumption of bone calcium, osteoporosis, liver and kidney fatigue, calculosis, and the consequent hypocalcemia, with all the results we have mentioned. It is appropriate to say, "*I eat less calcium to get more*".

Sodium and Potassium

In our organism *sodium* is generally found in its cation form, Na+, and in particular, it is the major cation that can be found in extracellular fluids.

Its concentration in the cell cytoplasm is insignificant. Its best-known role is linked to maintaining the body's water quota. One of the most common means of intake is in the form of a salt, NaCl. Its content in the body is regulated at the renal level through the action of a series of hormones, including *aldosterone*.

Also, as we read for calcium, it needs careful regulation. *Hyponatremia*, ie sodium deficiency, caused, for example, by an excess of water, not followed by the proper intake of the cation, leads to mental confusion, lethargy, neuromuscular hyper-excitability, up, in severe cases, to convulsions, coma and death. *Hypernatremia*, on the other hand, due to the loss of large quantities of water, sweating, unaccompanied by the loss of the cation, leads to thirst, alteration of brain function, confusional state, and again neuromuscular hyper-excitability, convulsions and coma. All in all, the results are the same.

Potassium is also found in our organism as a cation, K+, and represents the cation with the highest intracellular concentration. Unlike sodium, however, its reserves in the body are kept rather poor, so it needs more attention from the food point of view.

The maintenance of intracellular osmolality (concentration of a solution) is only one of its roles, but not the most important. In fact, it has important metabolic functions at the level of some enzymatic processes, but, above all, it participates in the excitability mechanism of nerve cells, in particular it has a direct role on the rhythm and contractility of the cardiac tissue; but we will discuss the topic in a moment. First I want to talk to you about the effects of concentration on the organism. *Hypokalaemia* due to vomiting, diarrhea or hormonal dysfunction, brings with it disturbances to the nervous, muscular and cardiac systems. *hyperkalemia*, caused by too high intracellular concentrations, due for example to renal failure, has clinical effects mainly on the myocardium, bradycardia, asystole and finally, cardiac arrest.

It is evident that the disorders of the organism, in case of wrong control of the sodium and potassium concentrations, are very similar. They are all mainly dependent on the nervous, musculoskeletal and cardiac systems. Obviously it is not a coincidence. It all depends on the indissoluble bond that the two cations have with the mechanism of the transmission of the electrical impulse, on the surface of the nerve cells and in particular on the bundles of neurites that make up the nerves and carry the orders of the brain anywhere in the body.

Said surface, in fact, has a negative electric charge, called *action potential*. In simple words, the impulse that is transmitted by the brain is nothing but a depolarization of this charge, which proceeds at a very high speed traveling the nerve fiber along its entire length. When the pulse arrives, the superficial negative charge decreases, the membrane then becomes permeable to the Na+ cations. These enter the cell and as they pass, the negative electrical potential collapses further, in turn depolarizing the neighboring region, at the starting point of the impulse.

From here it proceeds like a wave through the whole fiber. Once entered, the sodium cation is pumped immediately out of a system called "*Sodium-Potassium Pump*" which actively, that is, with energy consumption in the form of ATP, reports the concentration values to the initial levels, restoring the negative electrical potential of membrane. Every 2 ions of expelled sodium 3 of potassium are introduced into it.

At this point it is clear how the concentrations of the two cations are fundamental for the correct functioning of the pump, in the absence of one or the other the mechanism is jammed and the transmission of the electrical impulse is blocked. Hence all the unfortunate consequences mentioned above. The sodium-potassium pump jam also interferes with the electrical impulse that regulates the heartbeat.

Others minerals

Discuss all the minerals, which in some way interact with the complex functioning of the living organism, is objectively impossible here.

We will therefore limit ourselves to small hints:

Iron: fundamental element in the structure of the heme hemoglobin group, with the task of transporting oxygen into the blood. Participates in carbohydrate metabolism and antibody production.

Chlorine: in association with sodium, with which it forms the salt cooking molecule, NaCl, helps to maintain ionic electro-neutrality. It plays an important function at the gastric level where, in the form of hydrochloric acid, HCl, contributes to the digestive functions.

Magnesium: participates in numerous enzymatic processes and helps maintain muscle tone.

Copper: plays many roles and is present throughout the body, participates in the synthesis of the heme group, melanin, phospholipids of the myelin membrane of nerve cells, RNA. It contributes to numerous enzymatic functions, muscle elasticity, healing processes and bone structure.

Zinc: strong antioxidant properties, allows the absorption of some vitamins, especially those of group B. It participates in the mechanisms of some digestive enzymes and linked to the elimination of alcohol. It is a component of insulin. It is important for the growth and development of reproductive organs and prostate functions.

Manganese: intervenes in some enzymatic reactions. It is important for the development of the skeleton and after giving birth, participates in the production of breast milk. It is a metabolic regulator of sex hormones and the nervous system.

Selenium: fights free radicals together with vitamins C and E, participates in the formation of thyroid hormones.

Each of these substances participates in numerous reactions, in an infinity of mechanisms, also very different from each other and apparently without anything in common.

Although trace elements may have concentrations in the scale of micro-grams, their functions are very important and their absence can prove to be lethal. On the other hand, it is useless, if not harmful, to force the level of concentration: these substances, in fact, in massive doses are revealed poisons. In recent years we have seen an uncontrolled increase in the supply of salt and mineral supplements.

Every day the media are bombarding us by listing our food shortages and recommending us to use tablets filled with inorganic minerals with the promise of an iron health, it is appropriate to say so. The market is ruthless, you know.

But perhaps it is not known that a few years ago, faced with excessive costs for the disposal of materials resulting from the processing of aluminum, a multinational company, which I will not name, following a nefarious agreement with some pharmaceutical companies, has decided that selenium should become a human food, turning a waste into a miracle product for our health. Man becomes a means for the disposal of toxic substances. Perhaps not a subtle but surely brilliant (or criminal?) trick.

Once again we find ourselves speechless in the face of the lack of respect that some men have towards the delicacy and value of life.

Once again we must learn or, better, re-learn to recognize the most suitable food for us in natural foods. Although the concentrations of nutrients in natural food may seem insignificant, we are certain that the best doses are always the best for our organism to derive the best benefit from it.

No excesses, no deficiencies = Equilibrium.

12 LIPIDS (OR FATS)

I have never believed in bans without reasons and the media are full of warnings and advice...

Perfect strangers claim the right to tell us what is good for us and what hurts us.

Many, in perfect good faith, tell us their truths, but often without allowing us to understand. They underestimate us, they think that the explanation is too complex, they think it can confuse us. So it is better to keep us ignorant and use strong words that affect our susceptibility. Unfortunately all this always gets the opposite effect. And now? In this chapter we have to deal with a very complex subject, but it is absolutely important.

Fat: a word with obvious negative connotations. The bogeyman used over the years to scare people. To direct our food choices, sometimes with the aim of helping us, others to sell us diet products that, in the long run, are perhaps worse than the evil they want to cure.

What are fats? Meanwhile, I begin to call them by their right name: *lipids*, from the Greek *lypos*, precisely, fat. They are organic compounds, widely diffused in nature, which make up one of the four main classes of organic compounds of biological interest, along with carbohydrates, proteins and nucleic acids. Lipids are very heterogeneous molecules, formed by chains, more or less composed, of carbon atoms, joined together with covalent bonds, simple or double.

To these chains, called fatty acids, we can find bound molecules of alcohols, phosphoric groups, proteins, carbohydrates, etc., etc. Lipids have as their common characteristic a marked *lipophilia* (hydrophobia), that is, in an aqueous environment, they tend to gather together forming *bubbles*, with the aim of minimising the surface in contact with water. Another important feature of lipids is their melting point, that is, the variation in density at various temperatures. We will see in the following how both these characteristics can more or less change according to the complexity of the structures and what the consequences are.

Fatty acids are carbon chains, called *aliphatic*, which have at one end a carboxylic group, -COOH (fig.1).

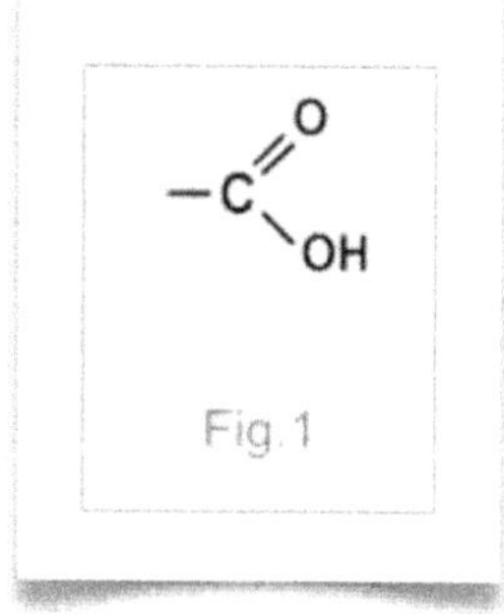

Fig. 1

In the images on the right we can see three examples of fatty acids: *saturated* (Fig. 2.1), ie without double covalent bonds, *monounsaturated* (Fig. 2.2), ie with only one double bond, and *polyunsaturated* (Fig. 2.3), with more than a double bond.

The oxygen atoms of the carboxylic group have a con-

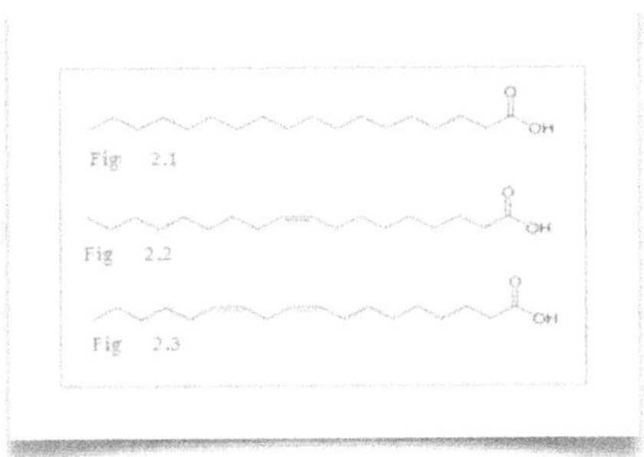

siderably larger diameter than the carbon atoms in the chain, so the electrons, which form a cloud that envelops the molecule, take longer to turn around the group. This fact generates a discrepancy of the negative electrical charge carried by the electrons.

The carboxylic group, therefore, constitutes a head in the chain, endowed with a slight negative charge, which is defined as *polar*. All this explains why in an aqueous solution the fatty acids tend to cluster in drops, with the polar heads, hydrophilic, towards the outside and the tails, apolar and lipophilic, towards the inside.

This conformation is called *Micella* (fig. 3).

The presence or absence of double bonds substantially modifies the shape of the carbon chains. As a result, the behavior of fatty acids also changes. These are called

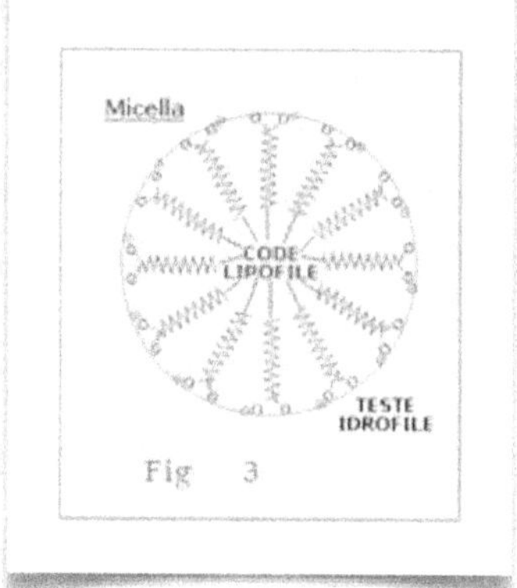

saturated, when the chains do not have double bonds. As we can see (fig.4) in the figure, the molecule turns out to

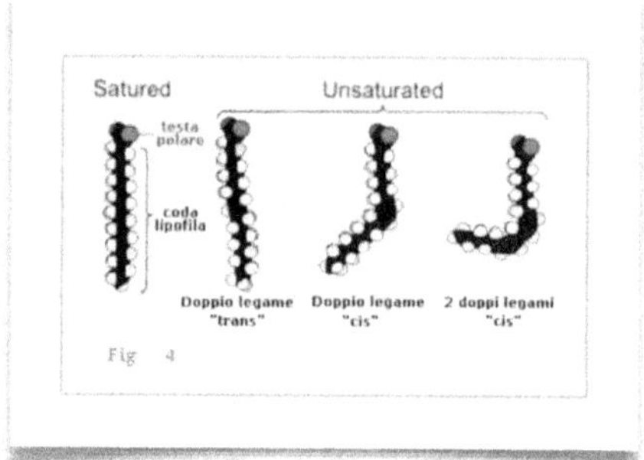

be rectilinear.

This arrangement allows the chains to overlap neatly, then at room temperature the lipid formed by saturated chains is in a solid state. This is a very frequent physical form in butter, lard and animal fats, whose structure has a higher percentage of saturated aliphatic chains. The presence of a double bond complicates things a bit. In fact, depending on how the hydrogen (H) atoms are arranged around the bond between the carbon atoms (C), the shape of the chain is modified. To get a clearer idea, let's look at figure 5.

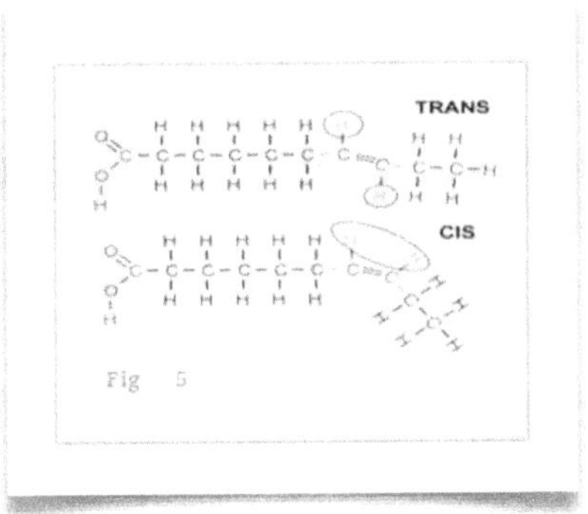

In the molecule shown in the figure, the two hydrogen atoms are located at opposite ends of the chain, TRANS layout. The lower molecule, on the other hand, shows the two hydrogens on the same side of the chain, CIS layout. All this is very important, because the different angles assumed by the bond significantly change the shape of the chain and its physical characteristics. In the first example, Trans, the chain is almost straight, in the second example, Cis, instead, has an angle of about 120°. It is evident that the presence of such distortions and angles in the chain prevent the ordered layout, typical of saturated chains.

The thing becomes even more evident in the presence of two or more double bonds. The chain will assume the most varied forms, depending on the layout and the atomic conformation of the double bonds.

This is the typical situation of vegetable oils, composed mostly of lipids whose unsaturated chains prevent an ordered layout. These oils, as everyone knows, at room temperature are in a liquid state.

However, the most common lipids are not formed from a single chain of fatty acid, but from aggregates of fatty acids and other substances. Thus, in living organisms, the most frequent lipidic charge is constituted by triglycerides (fig. 6), in which three fatty acid molecules join a glycerol molecule.

Depending on the types of aliphatic chains present, satu-

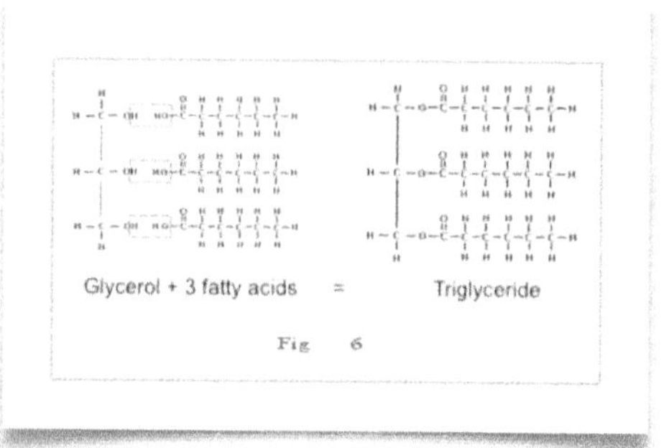

Fig   6

rated or otherwise unsaturated, we will have solid fats, such as butter, or liquids, such as olive oil. In nature, triglycerides and, more generally, lipids, present Cis aliphatic chains, which, I recall, have hydrogen atoms on the same side of the chain with respect to the double bond. This is very important because it directly affects our nutrition and consequently our health. In fact, unsaturated fats are more difficult to preserve, having a tendency to oxidise over time. Oxygen splits the double bond radically changing the chemical and organoleptic characteristics of the oils, which acidify.

The industry thought it was a good idea to saturate the oils with hydrogen atoms, a process that takes the name of hydrogenation. If the reader has a moment of time and the desire to do it, it is fun and a little alarming to browse through the ingredients of snacks and various industrial sweets. Hydrogenated fats are the masters. By saturating the aliphatic chains, these are straightened and can be arranged neatly like saturated fats of animal origin, so at room temperature, they are solid like butter. This is the case of margarine, for example. Moreover the saturation of the double bonds makes the fat, thus obtained, more resistant to oxidation and more durable over time.

These are excellent reasons to hydrogenate oils, according to the food industry, but for human health perhaps they are not as convincing. In fact, hydrogenation at high temperatures and strong pressures is not a natural process, and the result is substances that do not exist in nature. This is due to the fact that in living organisms the CIS or TRANS conformation of the aliphatic chains is decided and controlled by enzymes. As it happens, natural enzymes produce only CIS chains, with hydrogen on the same side.

Industrial hydrogenation, on the other hand, produces TRANS chains. No one, obviously, has wondered whether to insert substances that are not naturally present in such food can in some way hurt.

Or worse yet, maybe that someone has seen in this industrial process a way to use oils of extremely low quality, disguising them in synthetic fats and stuffing our food. Scientific research has actually already answered both our doubts. The use of hydrogenated fats, and in particular the intake of TRANS fatty acids, stimulates our liver to the massive synthesis of "bad cholesterol" (LDL lipoprotein), accompanied by a decrease in the synthesis of "good cholesterol" (HDL lipoprotein) , with all the harmful consequences that this can bring: for example, serious cardiovascular diseases (atherosclerosis, thrombosis, stroke, etc.). But of all this we will deal only in the remainder of the chapter.

One more little note.

In the stomach of cattle, there are bacteria that produce TRANS fatty acids. These are absorbed by the host organism and then poured into the cow's milk. We have already discussed in the chapter on the differences between human milk and cow's milk, here we have further confirmation of its dangerousness.

At this point we try to put a little 'order on the various types of lipids found in nature.

I can group the three large families of lipids:

- SIMPLE LIPIDS: Triglycerides (glycerol plus fatty acids)

- COMPOUND LIPIDS: Phospholipids and lipoproteins
- DERIVATIVE LIPIDS: Cholesterol

Simple lipids are mainly made up of triglycerides we have already discussed. They represent 95% of body fats. As we have seen, based on the concentration of saturated or otherwise unsaturated fatty acids, simple lipids can be in the solid or liquid state at room temperature.

Saturated fats are typically animals, like butter. Fish are the exception, especially those that inhabit cold seas, which are instead rich in polyunsaturated fats (Omega-3).

The explanation is very simple: the subcutaneous fat that covers these fish has a function of thermoregulation. If, at the ambient temperature close to 0° C, the fat became solid, they would no longer be able to swim, they would become rigid. Here is that mother nature has thought of the best system. The unsaturated fats form a gelatinous mass, soft and elastic even at the most rigid temperatures, allowing the fish to move easily.

The plant world, on the other hand, is rich in polyunsaturated fats, in the form of liquid oils.

The main function of triglycerides is to provide energy to the body, about 9 Kcal per gram. They also provide the fatty acids necessary for the various metabolic functions and those that are called essential fatty acids, ie that our body cannot synthesise itself, but must necessarily procure itself with food. These are polyunsaturated fatty acids and belong to two main categories, based on the position of the first double bond: Omega-3 (*α-linolenic* 18: 3) and Omega-6 (*alpha-linoleic* acid 18: 2). *Arachidonic* acid (20: 4), synthesized from linoleic acid, is the precursor of prostaglandins, whose task is to stimulate muscle cell contracture and to modulate cell responses to certain types of stimuli; *thromboxanes* and *leukotrienes*, very important chemical mediators involved in inflammation and platelet aggregation.

At this point we must make a distinction. The food industry has in recent years bombarded public opinion with a media campaign with the health goal of increasing consumption of Omega-3 fatty acids. In fact, according to research whose truthfulness and accuracy are out of the question, they have multiple positive actions on our body. Omega-3 lower plasma levels of triglycerides, interfering with the synthesis of VLDL lipoproteins (we'll see later what they are) in the liver; they have a modest hypo-cholesterolemic action; exert a positive action on the synthesis of cholesterol called "good", HDL lipoprotein; they are precursors of complex molecules that decrease the aggregation of platelets, with the consequent benefit on blood fluidity and the risk of coronary diseases; exert an anti-atherogenic, anti-inflammatory and anti-thrombotic action.

In the face of all these benefits, however, the media put the fish as the sole acidce of nourishment for the Omega-3s. The fish industry thanks, sardines and anchovies, on the verge of extinction, a little less.

And we, too, should not be thankful. The benefits deriving from the intake of Omega-3 from animal acidces, in fact, are inferior to the consequences of a diet rich in animal proteins and saturated acids, not absent in fish, as we have many time repeated in our book.

Also, I would like to dispel a little myth: if it is true that the Nordic fish are rich in unsaturated fats, it is not so true for those fish that come to our tables thanks to breeding.

In fact, to accelerate their growth, the latter are often fed with animal food rich in saturated fats; this involves a drastic drop in the percentages of unsaturated acids compared to saturated acids. As for Omega-6, however, the dietary benefits are very related to the amount taken with food. In fact, they have a good action on lowering the levels of "bad" cholesterol (LDL lipoprotein), but a modest effect on HDL; moreover, they have a low efficacy on the plasma concentrations of triglycerides; therefore, with few benefits, they have significant negative effects if taken in excess of Omega-3, such as the increase in allergic, inflammatory and blood pressure reactions; effects on platelet aggregation with risky cardiovascular consequences.

Attention, therefore, to excessive acidces of unsaturated Omega-6 acids, such as soy lecithin. These fats are definitely essential, but their intake in massive doses, compared to Omega-3, has significant effects on our health.

Another function of great importance of simple lipids is the protective one. Triglycerides, in fact, form fat deposits in the main organs, such as, for example, heart, liver, kidney, spleen, brain and spinal cord, so as to protect them from mechanical aggression. Finally, the layer of subcutaneous fat that covers our bodies has the function of reducing the heat loss through the epidermis. Attention, however, that precisely because of a diet too rich in fats, typical of our society, in these deposits the accumulation of triglycerides becomes excessive. Our mobility is compromised and the organs themselves are prevented by this informal mass in their principal functions.

In addition, an excess of fat mass proves to be just an obstacle to thermoregulation.

The compound lipids derive from the union of aliphatic chains to other substances, such as phosphoric groups (*phospholipids*), proteins (*lipoproteins*), carbohydrates (*glycolipids*) and others.

Phospholipids are among the most important, being a fundamental structural part of all cell membranes, from bacteria to superior life forms. They consist of two lipid, *lipophilic* tails, joined together with a head, the phosphoric, polar and hydrophilic group. This conformation, in an aqueous environment, as we have already explained for single-chain fatty acids, pushes the phospholipids to aggregate into bifilar structures with the heads facing the water and the tails facing inwards. Thus, an impermeable, spherical membrane is formed, with water both outside and inside, in two separate environments.

This structure, of greatest importance for life, is naturally formed as a result of the conformation of the phospholipids itself, without any external action.

Lipids are insoluble in water, which makes it impossible to transport them dissolved into the blood plasma. At this point, the need arises, to transport them in the body, to bind them to other molecules (*carriers*), in particular proteins, to make them soluble.

Complex molecules are thus formed, known as lipoproteins, which are divided into groups according to their chemical properties: the *chylomicrons* are formed in the intestinal walls, with the aim of collecting and transporting lipids from the digestion into the lymphatic ducts.

They consist mainly of triglycerides and only minimally of cholesterol and phospholipids. Through the circulation they are transferred to the liver which metabolize them and transforms them to be stored in the form of fat deposits. Another important function is the transport of some liposoluble, lipid-based vitamins, such as A, D, E, K.

High-density lipoproteins (HDL), produced in the liver and intestines, have the ability to remove cholesterol from the arterial walls to transport it to the liver, where it is used for biliary synthesis. For this reason they are sometimes called "*good cholesterol*". The importance of these lipoproteins for our arterial health is evident.

Finally, low density lipoproteins (LDL) and very low density (VLDL), consisting essentially of lipids and cholesterol and to a lesser extent proteins. LDL lipoproteins, near the cells of the arterial endothelium, release the cholesterol they carry.

This attaches to the vessel wall and stimulates cell proliferation at the point of attachment. It follows a narrowing of the lumen of the vessel, which compromises the ability to pass the blood. In a first phase, this involves an increase in blood pressure, necessary for the blood to reach all the regions, then, as the tissue continues to grow, there is the occlusion of the vessel. This thing does not generally have serious consequences: considering that the various regions of the organism are reached by many vessels and capillaries, the inefficiency of one of them does not compromise the functionality, that of very small portions of them. Unfortunately, and there is always a unfortunately, the circulatory system of the heart, which we normally know as the coronary system, has a peculiar characteristic: the ramifications of the vessels that supply the heart muscle are few and not intersected with each other. This means that when one of the vessels closes, the compromised region is quite extensive.

The lack of oxygenation of the tissues quickly leads to necrosis and death of the tissue itself, which, when it comes to heart muscle, means heart attack and / or premature death of the individual. Also cerebral circulation presents similar risks. It is absolutely necessary to avoid the proliferation of these occluding deposits, because once created, their elimination also presents great risks. The most common methods for recovering vessel function are *surgical*.

The famous coronary By-passes or the use of balloon probes, which once threaded and inflated, force the vessels to reopen. During these operations, however, and in the following days, the mechanically stressed cholesterol deposits release fragments of fat and tissue that enter the blood bed.

A consequence, unfortunately very frequent, is that these fragments reach the cerebral circulation, occlude an important vessel, leading to the onset of a cerebral stroke, with all the terrible consequences that it entails. The medical literature reports that the percentage of stroke in individuals who have recently undergone coronary interventions is very high for the whole of the following year. It is something to really meditate on, in front of a plate of succulent grilled pork ribs.

The family of derived lipids, just as the name implies, is made up of substances derived from simple and composed lipids. The most important exponent of this class is *cholesterol*.

Cholesterol is a *sterol*, that is, a steroid with an alcohol function in position 3, those wishing to deepen can consult organic chemistry texts.

Cholesterol is synthesized at the liver level; It is meant then of endogenous cholesterol. Despite all the bad publicity that has been done by the media, it is essential for the life of our body. In addition to being a very important component of cell membrane structure, cholesterol is necessary for the synthesis of multiple steroid-based compounds, such as bile salts, adrenal hormones, androgens, estrogens and progesterone. Furthermore, it is a precursor of vitamin D.

Cholesterol can also be taken with digestion, exogenously, and there is an inverse relationship between endogenous synthesis and exogenous intake. This means that even in a low-cholesterol diet, our body produces the amount it needs. Unfortunately, if the diet is too rich, the body is not as efficient in its elimination, with all the negative effects already described.

Cholesterolemia, that is, the levels of cholesterol in the blood, is very variable from individual to individual, and subject to variations related to the diet. In fact, the intake of saturated fats stimulates the synthesis, while the intake of unsaturated and polyunsaturated fats, except TRANS fats, decreases their blood levels.

Also the contribution of fibers, decreasing the absorption of bile salts by the intestine, has as an indirect consequence the decrease in blood cholesterol levels. Finally, there are substances in nature that can compete with cholesterol at the level of receptors and intestinal absorption. These take the name of *phytosterols*, among which one very active is *beta phytosterol*. The extra virgin olive oil, if poorly worked and refined, has good levels of phytosterols.

To conclude, that of lipids is a rich and complex topic. They are fully among the most important substances for life and come into play in many functions and reactions of the organism.

Cell membranes, energy, protection, the synthesis of many hormones, vitamins ... All this shows us how much each piece of the puzzle is important, and once again it is evident how a reckless diet can transform a class of molecules, absolutely necessary for life, in poison. As always, we must learn that the balances are fundamental and very delicate and that we must take control of what we eat to guarantee our health.

In other chapters of this book we can find out what foods can best help us in our pursuit of health and ultimately, of happiness.

On the market there are slimming phytosanitary products able to intercept lipids at the level of intestinal absorption. It is impossible to deny its effectiveness in a generalist diet based on large quantities of animal fats, but beware: as we have discovered, many vitamins are lipid-based or have some precursors in lipids.

These slimmers, even though they have almost no contraindications in the warning sheet, also intercept this class of substances. Vitamin deficiency following weight loss can nullify the benefits of the diet.

The supplementary intake of synthetic vitamins is practically nil. Once again, respect for one's own body must take place upstream.

Vegetarian diets, possibly vegan, better raw food, best Natural Diet, will be the right basis to regain control of your body, return to love it and above all restore the biological balance necessary for a healthy and vigorous life.

13 OMEGA-3

In 2010 in Great Britain, scientific research was carried out, later published in the *American Journal of Clinical Nutrition*: about 20,000 people were involved in carrying out this study. Research shows that the absorption of Omega-3 is much more efficient if of plant origin. During this research it emerged that individuals who follow a strict vegetarian diet, ie excluding any animal products, including fish, are able to derive the long chain Omega-3 (present in fish products) from Omega-fatty acids 3 plants; these fats are important for the body's metabolic functions and can be introduced through the plant diet without resorting to fish intake.

For those seriously dealing with nutrition, the result of this research is not seen as a novelty but simply as a confirmation. It has been known for some time now that Omega-3s are more easily assimilated from a plant-based diet than from a fish-based diet, as most people mistakenly believe.

The fish, moreover, contains Omega-3 in quantities much less than is believed, since with cooking, these fatty acids decrease considerably.

This new research is another confirmation of how the privileged acidce of Omega-3 is precisely that found in foods of plant origin.

Before exposing the results of other researches, we clarify to better understand what the Omega-3 are: the *PUFA N3* (Omega-3) are polyunsaturated fatty acids, known for their fundamental role of cell maintenance and integrity.

The most important fatty acids of the Omega-3 group are three: *α-linolenic acid* (Anglo-Saxon abbreviation *ALA*), *eicosapentaenoic acid (EPA)* and *docosahexaenoic acid (DHA)*. ALA are "short chain" Omega-3 and are found in vegetables, in green leafy vegetables (mostly in spinach) and more abundantly in nuts and seeds; EPAs and DHAs are "long chain" Omega-3s and they are most needed by the cells; they are found in fish products, algae and eggs made from hens fed on a diet rich in fish.

The human body needs EPA and DHA essentially for the cells, the brain, the immune system and all metabolic functions. Some small clinical studies have suggested that humans can convert only small percentages of Omega-3 EPA and DHA, necessary for their health, from Omega-3 ALA from plant foods.

As a result, these researchers, in agreement with the health authorities, have considered smarter to obtain EPA and DHA directly through fish intake. For these reasons the FDA has approved the intake of Omega-3 only from foods or supplements that contain EPA and DHA or only DHA. It also authorised milk producers to enrich it with Omega-3 DHA. This is probably why most nutritionists, aligned with health authorities, promote fish based diets, claiming that it is the only way to get benefits from Omega-3 (EPA and DHA). The hypothesis, that only fish products could provide EPA and DHA to humans, was denied by clinical analysis performed on adults who grew up observing a strictly vegan diet.

A British study shows that the organism of vegan people adapts to the lack of fats deriving from fish, increasing the conversion speed in EPA and DHA from the Omega-3s taken with vegetables (ALA). The same British team has recently published a larger study confirming the hypothesis that the organism is able to produce EPA and DHA from the Omega-3 ALA in more than sufficient quantities: it was found a greater production than previously thought.

The researchers found in the blood of the individuals examined, less difference than expected of EPA and DHA, despite the great differences in their intake of Omega-3, derived from the different diet.

The new findings come from a research group led by Ailsa Welch at the *British University of East Anglia*. Previously there were small metabolic studies, aimed at determining the degree of conversion of ALA into EPA and DHA, but this appears to be the first study carried out on a large population with different eating habits. What the British study has shown is summarized here: the subjects of the study were 14,422 men and women between the ages of thirty-nine and seventy-eight, all participating in a cancer risk survey; thereafter, 4,902 people were selected who had been tested for the blood level of fatty acids.

Doctor Welch and his collaborators subdivided the individuals into "*fish eaters*", "*carnivores except fish*", *vegetarians* and *vegans*, comparing the respective blood values of ALA, EPA and DHA.

Fish eaters took 57 to 80% more Omega-3s of their diet than those who followed fish-free diets, but the differences in blood levels of DHA and EPA in the four groups of people were minimal. The level of EPA for those who fed on fish was 64.7 micromoles (μmol) per liter compared to 57 (μmol) in carnivores, 55 (μmol) in vegetarians and 50 (μmol) in vegans. Meanwhile, the average level of DHA found was 271 (μmol) for those who ate fish, 241 (μmol) for carnivores, 223 (μmol) for vegetarians and an even higher value of 286 (μmol) for vegans.

This study also confirms the results of past research that showed a higher conversion of ALA in EPA and DHA in women, compared to men and higher conversion rates in "non-fish eaters" compared to those who include fish products in their own diet.

This research thus shows that, despite the great difference between diets with or without fish-based meals, the values of useful Omega-3, ie EPA and DHA found in plasma, are almost the same, with such small differences that induce scientists to believe that the greatest conversion occurs precisely between those who do not directly take EPA and DHA from food, but transform them from ALA contained in vegetables.

It is therefore useless to eat fish meat to get the Omega-3 needed, better to resort to alternative and healthy acidces such as vegetables.

Other studies warn about the use of Omega-3 supplements: Omega-3 fatty acids derived from fish (DHA and EPA) are often sold as fish oil capsule supplements, but recently some researchers have "discovered" that they are not as healthy as many believe and indeed, they are extremely harmful to our health.

A study published in the *American Journal of Epidemiology* conducted by dr. Theodore M. Brasky (Seattle, USA 2011) has shown that individuals with a higher blood value of DHA are more at risk of incurring prostate cancer. The research was carried out by examining 3,461 patients during a study for the prevention of prostate cancer: among the individuals examined it was discovered that those who ate fish or took Omega-3 supplements, were up to two and a half times more at risk of developing the tumor to the prostate; the higher the level of DHA in the blood, the greater the risk of prostate cancer.

Other studies have denied the advertised "benefits of fish oil". In fact, such research has never had serious feedback on the supposed benefits.

No "miracle" promised by an Omega-3 supplement has ever been scientifically proven since this capsule does not help heart patients, does not help treat or prevent Alzheimer's disease, does not fight depression and does not seem to enhance intelligence in children.

In 2005, in the Journal of the *American Medical Association (JAMA)*, an article appeared on a study that revealed that the supposed benefit against cardiac arrhythmia, caused by the consumption of fish oil, was non-existent, on the contrary it was found that in some patients its use worsened the situation.

In 2006, the same magazine published a report of thirty-eight scientific studies concerning the relationship between Omega-3 fatty acids and cancer cases. All these research led to the same conclusion: fish oil is completely useless for the prevention of tumors. According to an analysis carried out in 2009 on five thousand individuals (*Rotterdam Study*), a diet rich in fish or supplements of EPA and DHA does not reduce in the least even the problems of heart failure.

Out of five thousand patients under medical supervision with myocardial infarction, there were no differences in new cardiovascular events among those who were prescribed the use of Omega-3 supplements and those who took a placebo: the details of this study can be find in an article published in 2010 on the *New England Journal of Medicine*.

Instead, the results of a study by Harvard School of Medicine researchers were surprising: in 2009 these scholars found a connection between consumption of fish or the use of Omega-3 EPA and DHA supplements, and type 2 diabetes.

Researchers analyzed 200,000 adults for about eighteen years, highlighting that among these, individuals who were affected by type 2 diabetes were the largest consumers of fish products or Omega-3 supplements (Kaushik, 2009). The producers of fish oil, in light of the new scientific data unfavorable to them, focused everything on the "intelligence" effect that this integrator would give.

In 2010, however, this unfounded belief was refuted by a subsequent study: during two years of analysis on 867 elderly, half of them was given an oil supplement containing DHA and EPA, while the other half was given a placebo based on olive oil; at the end of the long observation period, no difference was found in terms of cognitive functions between the two groups of patients.

There are many studies on the subject and still in development, but all have the same results.

The human being is able to produce the useful Omega-3 (DHA and EPA) from plant foods and this mechanism helps the body to autonomously regulate the quantity of fatty acids according to its needs, without having to suffer the damages caused by an excess of DHA and EPA that, as shown, besides being inefficient in preventing the onset of diseases, often favour them.

14 CARBOHYDRATES

Sugars, starches, fibers, glucides, saccharides …
In the following pages I will try to put some order in this confusion of chemicals, because knowledge gives us the ability to choose the best and to defend ourselves from those who exploit ignorance and misunderstanding for purposes far from our well-being.

Carbohydrate implies a chain of hydrated carbon atoms, but the class of organic substances we will talk about is more varied and complex. The Italian word "glucidi" comes from the Greek "*glucos*" = sweet.

As said for proteins and lipids, these compounds are formed by cyclic chains, that is formed by aggregation of several base units, the *monosaccharides*, in turn formed by carbon and hydrogen chains joined to alde-hyde groups (aldehydes, see figure 7)

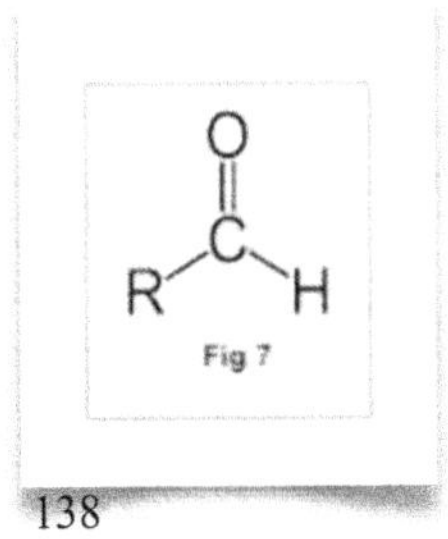

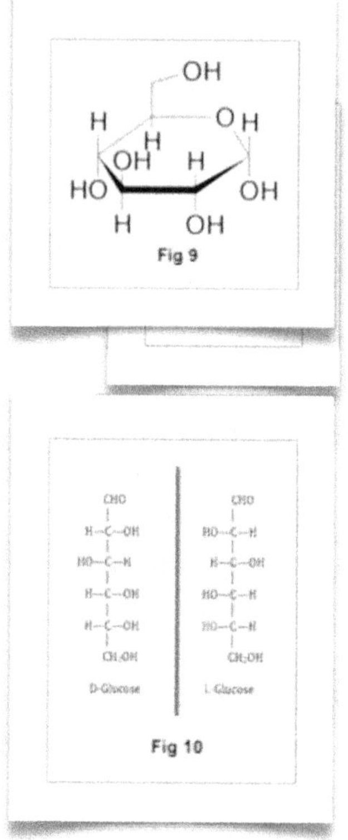

Fig 9

Fig 10

or ketones (ketones, figure 8).

In the two figures, the letters R and R' indicate generic carbon chains. Simple carbohydrates are made up of single monosaccharides which are generally in equilibrium in their open, linear, and closed-loop form, with a predominance of the second structure. The composed carbohydrates are formed by rings of monosaccharides joined together.

So, we have *monosaccharides*, *disaccharides*, with two rings of monosaccharides, *oligosaccharides*, when the rings are between 3 and 10 and *polysaccharides*, with more than 10 monosaccharides. Monosaccharides, as also happens in fatty acids, in aqueous solution can change the incidence of light in a clockwise or counter-clockwise direction.

This characteristic is due to the structure of the molecule when it is open. In fact, two identical forms can coexist, but one specular to the other, hence the name of dextro-rotatory or levorotatory molecule (Fig.9 - 10).

It is a characteristic that should not be underestimated, because if, even in appearance, the chemical qualities seem the same, in truth there are differences. Nature usually prefers one of the two forms. An example is glu-cose and fructose.

Both monosaccharides, both with 6 carbon atoms (*hex-ose*), the first derived from an aldehyde, then *aldose*, the latter from a ketone, *ketose*. Glucose in nature exists al-most exclusively in the dextrorotatory form, it is called *dextrose*; fructose, instead, in the levorotatory form, *lev-ulose*. This is due to the fact that, in nature, the creation of these molecules takes place with the help of enzymes whose synthesis is genetically regulated.

These enzymes only build dextrorotatory molecules for glucose and levorotatory for fructose. A bit like the keys that have only one lock that can open. A mirror key, de-spite having the same profile, is not able to open the lock of his image.

These asymmetries are often underestimated in the con-text of industrial synthesis, where some chemical pro-cesses used do not discern between the two chiral struc-tures.

So we are selling synthetic substitute products that do not respect what we could call "mother nature specifications" compromising our health. In fact, the enzymes involved in metabolic reactions are specific. Not recognizing the copies, I am not able to process them properly. The results are variable. We go from the complete inability to complete a cycle of reactions, to the most serious situation, in which the reactions are carried out only partially, with the formation of unexpected products that are easily harmful to health.

For human biology the most important monosaccharides are three: the already mentioned glucose and *fructose*, to which *galactose* is added. As we have said, these three can be linked together forming chains, ranging from two to several hundred monomers, giving rise to an infinity of glucose compounds.

Among the most important disaccharides are *sucrose*, formed by the union of glucose and fructose (cooking sugar), *lactose*, fundamental component of milk, from the union between glucose and galactose, and *maltose*, glucose combined with glucose.

The oligosaccharide class includes sugars such as *raffinose*, *stachyose* and *verbascose*, which cannot be digested by humans, composed of galactose, glucose and fructose, and mainly contained in legumes.

The production of gas, following the fermentation of these sugars in the large intestine, explains the meteorism caused, above all in some subjects, by the consumption of legume products.

The polysaccharides, as obvious, represent the largest group, thousands of compounds among which it is absolutely necessary to point out the *starch*, energy reserve of the plants, formed by very long chains of glucose and *glycogen*, energy reserve in the animal world, branched polymer formed by chains of glucose, just like its vegetable counterpart (fig.11).

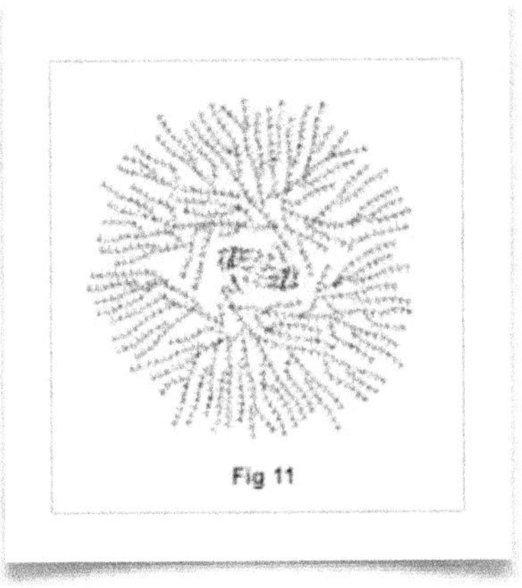

As we have just read together, starch is the preferred energy reserve in the plant world; the differences with glycogen are limited to the number of monomers, the size of the macromolecule and the complexity of the ramifications.

Starch provides longer lasting energy and for a longer period, characteristics that are well suited to the metabolism of a plant, but less suited to the liveliest and fastest metabolism of an animal; for this reason, the glycogen structure fits itself better to the needs of the latter. The starch, which we find in large quantities in bread, pasta, rice and potatoes, once ingested, is broken down into the glucose monomers.

Glucose passes the stomach walls very quickly, reaches the blood bed and, once reached the liver and striated muscle cells, is, if not used immediately, transformed into glycogen and stored.

The amount of glycogen used as a reserve is not really much; under physical stress it is quickly converted into simple and burned glucose, the autonomy is about twenty minutes. The excess of glucose, not transformed into glycogen, is converted to the liver in triglycerides and then all ends up on our flanks.

Once again we have to observe the details, because nature is very sensitive to these. The link between glucose monomers in starch is called *α-glycosidic*, due to its position within the carbon ring. There are various positions in the ring in which the bond can occur, and one in particular gives rise to a bond called *β-glycosidic*. I do not want to exaggerate, entering further into the organic chemistry of these elements, but only to point out to you that, by simply moving the link from position α to β, starch turns into cellulose. Fundamental element in the structure of the cell walls of plants and completely indigestible to humans. In fact, we possess the α-amylase enzymes in the intestine, not the β-amylases. How many times have we been told, now we have understood why.

Only some ruminants possess in their stomach a bacterial flora capable of digesting cellulose.

At this point we have understood that the class of glucose compounds, called carbohydrates, is rich and really varied. They carry out numerous biological functions, including energy reserve and transport (for example starch and glycogen) or as structural components of cellulose in plants and cartilage in animals. Furthermore, they play a fundamental role in the immune system, in fertility and in biological development.

How can we not emphasize that *ribose* and *deoxyribose*, two carbohydrates, are fundamental components of RNA and DNA, the very foundations of our life?

Glucose certainly deserves a more detailed mention. It is, of course, in its dextrorotatory form called *dextrose*, the most abundant monosaccharide in nature. Produced by plants in the process of photosynthesis, it certainly plays a very important role in the energetic metabolism of living beings and of man. The oxidative combustion of glucose provides about 4 Kcal / gr, therefore slightly less than half of the lipids, but given its ability to quickly pass cell membranes, to cross the stomach walls, to be transported quickly into the bloodstream to effectively reach all the interstices of the organism, the ease of energy storage in the form of glycogen and, finally, its stability and minimum reactivity towards proteins and other compounds, all these things make it an exceptional compound in the body. So much so that the nervous system draws the energy it needs only from glucose.

The energetic process begins with *glycolysis*, i.e. the cleavage of the glucose molecule. This first step gives rise to pyruvic acid, because of two molecules for each glucose molecule consumed, plus 2 molecules of ATP, a true cell energy vector.

At this point, in the presence and consumption of oxygen, the process continues in what is called the "*cycle of*

Krebs" or oxidative respiration, which results in carbon dioxide, water and as many as 26 molecules of ATP which, with the addition of the previous 2, brings the total to 28. In the event of lack of oxygen the reactions continue in the anaerobic respiration, which results in the formation of lactic acid and a rather low energy yield.

During intense physical exertion, the consumption of oxygen, to complete the oxidative respiration and to support a greater energy demand by the muscular tissues, increases rapidly.

The demand for air increases, so breathing becomes more frequent and deeper. If, however, the effort continues, it happens that in some regions of the muscle, oxygen does not reach the sufficient quantity. This blocks the Krebs cycle and initiates anaerobic fermentation. Muscle efficiency decreases and lactic acid accumulates in the tissues.

At this point, muscle pains and cramps arise which, even when the effort is over, will continue for a few days, until the acid is completely disposed of.

As we said, glycogen stores do not have a very prolonged duration under stress. Once exhausted, following a continuous glucose request, the organism will be forced to operate reactions able to produce it starting from proteins and lipids. This mechanism is called *glu-coneogenesis* and occurs mainly in the liver.

Blood glucose levels are of utmost importance. The brain is not able to produce energy from other compounds and is very sensitive even to the smallest variations. Blood sugar, the name given to the concentration of glucose in the blood, must

always be under strict regulation by the body. The hormones insulin and glucagon, both produced in the pancreatic islets of Langerhans, are concerned with maintaining blood glucose levels in the right range.

I have already discussed previously the topics related to various diseases, among which diabetes is definitely the protagonist. Here I will limit myself to saying that a blood glucose deficiency (*hypoglycemia*) brings a general sense of weakness, accompanied by other symptoms such as pallor, palpitations, sialorrhea, tremors, etc.

A persistent *hyperglycemia* over time leads to very severe symptoms: intense thirst, tiredness, increased urination frequency and amount of urine, visual disturbances, cramps, smell of acetone in breath, nausea, vomiting, neurological changes up to coma.

Glucose is the glucide that stimulates the variation of the blood glucose level with greater intensity and speed. For this reason, it acts as a reference point for defining the glycemic index, which, in simple terms, is a number that describes the rate at which glucose increases following the intake of 50 g of any glucide. Given the glucose index (50 g) equal to 100, we can build a scale for all the others. To give an example, an index of 50 tells us that the glucide (50gr) raises the blood sugar to half the rate of glucose.

All this to introduce another very important actor in this endless plot that is life, *fructose*. I have already mentioned this, now we have to talk about it in depth. I summarize the characteristics: fructose is a monosaccharide with six carbon atoms (*hexose*), very similar then to glucose, but unlike this, as we have already seen, comes from a ketone.

In nature it exists almost exclusively in the levorotatory (*levulose*) structure, but it can be synthesized in the laboratories in the dextrorotatory form (very used in the substitutive formulas for newborns, like "let's hurt ourselves"). Like glucose, too, it tends to close in a ring, this time pentagonal. A glucose and a fructose joined together form the disaccharide sucrose, the common cooking sugar.

Fructose is very common in the plant world. In fact, it is found in the overwhelming majority of sugary fruits, in honey and also in some vegetables. In the cane and in the sugar beet, it is found in low concentrations in its simple state, but, if we consider how these plants are rich in sucrose, we can understand that they too are an excellent acidce of this monosaccharide.

In relation to the glycemic index, fructose is the glucide with the lowest absolute index. A very important feature, considering a diet rich in fructose, then fruit, in correlation with some diseases such as diabetes.

Insulin is the hormone that has the task of breaking down blood sugar. A diet rich in fructose, given the glycemic index so low, affects much less the increase in blood sugar, so it is less sensitive to the inefficiency of insulin synthesis of a diabetes patient.

Blood sugar maintains correct values regardless of the ability to produce insulin. This explains why, many diabetics, even for a long time, report the decrease in insulin dosage from the moment they undertake a fruitarian diet. It is not a trivial matter, if we consider also a young and healthy individual who, through a diet rich in carbohydrates, puts for all his life the pancreatic isles under stress, in the face of an abundant production of insulin, necessary to balance the very high glycemic glucose index.

The research is based on observation. Researchers, therefore, when they study the mechanisms of human energy metabolism, are based on the data and characteristics of modern man. This situation, however, has generated a misunderstanding. As we have seen, glycolysis, the first step of oxidative respiration, begins, according to studies carried out by biochemists, with a glucose molecule and ends with the formation of two pyruvic acid molecules and 2 ATP. I wanted to leave this topic at the end of the discussion so as not to burden it too much and also to create a bit of surprise, but what I have not told you yet is that glucose, before being divided into two, is transformed, with consumption of 2 molecules of ATP, then energy, in fructose. Then it will be fructose, which in fact will be split from the reaction, to give the aforementioned products, plus 4 molecules of ATP. To recapitulate: glucose turns into fructose with consumption of 2 ATP; fructose is transformed into 2 pyruvates plus 4 ATP.

Energy result of the 2 ATP reaction (4-2 = 2). The organism of modern man, due to the very rich diet of carbohydrates and sugars, must dispose of an incredible quantity of glucose. Fructose is relegated to a corner. As always, our body, in the presence of the scarcity of the substances it needs, turns to reactions that can keep it alive and that can make up for that lack.

In short, for many years, that is, since man had to abandon the fruit-based diet rich in fructose, due to climatic upheavals, we lived in a state of emergency, replacing fructose with glucose, of which the new diet was very rich.

An emergency that still lasts today. An emergency that researchers have turned into a rule. Why convert glucose into fructose, with energy expenditure, when we could simply use the second one, with a double energy yield? Second point. During an intense physical effort, with great energy expenditure, we will have to face a high consumption of ATP, necessary for muscle contraction. Glucose glycolysis, to begin with, needs 2 ATP and, in the situation described above, these are poor, the reaction slows down and a vicious circle is created: greater ATP demand to satisfy muscular effort, lower cell capacity producing it, due to its lack precisely in the initial phase of the reaction. This situation explains very clearly the increase in sports performance, associated with many studies in the fruitarian diet.

Fructose does not need to consume ATP in glycolysis, compared to a quadruple energy yield (4-0 = 4). The reaction does not slow down due to the lack of ATP, the **Krebs** cycle can continue with maximum efficiency. Speaking of glucose we have described its easy transportability through cell membranes and then through the blood.

All this is true, so much so that the glucose passes immediately the stomach walls and, following its ingestion, it reaches the blood bed immediately. The point is that the mechanisms of glucose transport are active, ie they require energy, therefore, in the formula of the energy balance of glucose, we must also include this dispersed energy for its transport.

Once again this monosaccharide loses in its comparison with the fructose rival, able to cross the cell walls without the intervention of active pumps. The energy inefficiency of transport makes the energy balance strongly in favour of fructose; it is estimated that the energy difference can approach 1.5 times higher in favour of fructose. Glucose, with its aldehyde group, is essentially a derivative alcohol. In aqueous solution it is therefore acidifying. Fructose, derived from a ketone, has no effect on the acid-base balance of the organism. I refer the reader to the chapter concerning the acidity of the organism and its consequences and I limit myself to say that if we add to the formula of the energy balance of glucose the energy necessary to buffer its acidity, the gap between the yields of the two monosaccharides becomes incredibly wide: about 13 times greater in favour of fructose.

What do we get from all this? We can state that glucose, due to its stability and, since it is naturally formed without the need for enzymes, is a very old fuel. Perhaps the first used by the forms of life appeared on earth. With the arrival of fruit trees, however, things have changed. Fructose, for its energy efficiency, has outclassed and replaced glucose in its energy leadership. Man, in his frugivorous nature, has drawn from this monosaccharide all the evolutionary advantages. But, in an unfortunate historical moment, he had to change his diet to survive the famine. Since then, he has not been able to go back, continuing to live in a constant state of emergency.

Of all the fruits present on the planet, the apple has fructose concentrations close to 92% of the carbohydrates of which it is made. This certainly makes it one of the most complete fruits. It is no coincidence, if the estimated place of origin of the apple is the African continent, in the area of the great lakes between Kenya and Zaire, considered the cradle of man's origin.

The voices against.

In recent years it has been discovered that fructose has many industrial advantages. Its extraction from corn syrups is not expensive, compared to the production of sugar cane or beet. Furthermore, the sweetening power of fructose exceeds that of glucose by a good 30%. It means that, to get the same sensation of sweetness on the palate, (even if the taste buds are found on the tongue) we can use a much lower dose of fructose than glucose. For the industry this is godsend.

We can see that fructose quickly gained the upper hand as a sweetener in almost all industrial desserts and drinks. Ingested doses quickly became high, then too high and finally excessive. At this point, some research laboratories (perhaps subsidised by producers of sucrose), have wondered if fructose can hurt.

So, it was thought to take guinea pigs, feed them for weeks with massive doses of fructose and then watch how they get by. Well, they did not get along well. Fructose in these conditions is harmful for the guinea pigs and probably also for the man.

We must move away from these market logic and at least ambiguous science. Refined fructose, ingested in large quantities, is certainly lethal, as is water and the same oxygen if we exaggerate with them. Nothing comparable to fructose ingested with fruit.

To ingest a pure and refined fructose etc, how many kilos of fruit should I swallow? Moreover, with fructose in fruit there are many useful substances: organic water, salts, vitamins, enzymes and last but not least the fibers. In fact, given our inability to digest them, they play a fundamental role. The rate of absorption of the intestine slow down and this contributes enormously to avoiding the glycemic peaks resulting from nutrition.

Since the beginning of the last century fructose has been used as a substitute sweetener for people with diabetes and, for the reasons mentioned above, it has certainly been effective.

In recent years, however, synthetic sweeteners have made their way, such as saccharin and aspartame, which thanks to an almost zero caloric power and a sweetening power hundreds of times higher than glucose, have quickly conquered the market.

Unfortunately, as for all the substances synthesized and not present in nature, the voices of their faults for the development of cancers and tumors quickly made their way and the laboratory tests confirmed them. Attention therefore to the use of so-called "light" substances, which rage in the markets, in which the normal and natural sugars have been replaced by these sweeteners; they are potentially very harmful to health.

It is appropriate to say that the cure may be worse than the disease.

We have thus come to the end of a long chapter, perhaps a bit difficult, but that, given the importance of the argument, it was not possible to contain in a shorter space.

The conclusions are obvious: useless to demonize the carbs, basic compounds for our body and for life. As we will never tire of repeating, it will always and only be to maintain correct and balanced eating behaviors. Once again, the pieces of the puzzle have gone well and we have been able to discover together that all metabolic reactions are interdependent with each other, that varying the ingredients of the diet can radically change the effects on our well-being and life.

A diet based on fruit or at least very rich (especially apples) has incredible effects on our health, even in the presence of major diseases such as diabetes, significantly improving the quality of the years we still have to spend on this beautiful Earth.

15 HEME AND NOT HEME IRON

Iron is a fundamental mineral for the good functioning of the human body because it contributes to the formation of those substances that, through the blood flow, participate in the transport mechanisms of oxygen in all organs, tissues and cells.

The iron intake of those who follow vegetarian diets is often the cause of debate because some misinformed dieticians accuse the meatless diet of being the primary cause of a possible iron deficiency.

The majority of doctors and nutrition experts, "strangely" seem to be unaware of recent discoveries, and continue undaunted to argue that a diet comprising animal products is essential to prevent or treat iron deficiency. The same doctors, however, rightly admit the importance of foods rich in vitamin C as vegetables and fruit in general, because they consider them absolutely necessary for optimal assimilation of minerals, including iron.

Normally doctors and dietitians believe that the major acidces of iron and B vitamins are red meat and dairy products; they also claim that the iron contained in plants is less assimilable, advising the consumption of meat to combat anemia resulting from iron deficiency.

The arguments about the different degree of assimilability of iron of animal or vegetable origin may seem true only by observing very superficially the characteristics of iron coming from meat, called *heme iron*, and from iron of vegetable origin (present in vegetables, legumes, cereals and in fruit), called *non-heme iron*.

The iron of animal derivation (iron heme) is commonly considered superior to non-heme (of vegetable origin) in terms of bio-availability, but this is true only when the diet lacks an adequate supply of natural foods containing vitamin C (as fruit and vegetables). Hence, heme iron is more assimilable, but it is not suitable for the assimilative system of man because it has an effect that is too violent, traumatic and stimulating.

Anemia, ie a condition characterized by a decrease in the total amount of hemoglobin present in the body, is caused by multiple and complex factors and not only by nutritional deficiencies.

Some doctors and nutritionists claim that among vegetarians there is an increased risk of iron deficiency anemia, but recent research has categorically denied this assumption. In fact, it has been discovered that cases of anemia due to iron deficiency are equally present both in people following an omnivorous diet, and among those who prefer vegetarian diets.

Other data also show that vegans have a lower percentage of cases of anemia than lacto-ovo-vegetarians and non-vegetarians. In addition, those who follow vegetarian diets, despite having lower levels of iron deposit, have values of blood levels of ferritin absolutely normal. A low value of ferritin can mean both a diet low in iron and an excess of losses, due to causes such as hemorrhoids or very intense menstruation, but remember that the most important reason is the consumption of substances that limit the absorption of iron.

Anemia due to iron deficiency is very common, affecting 700 million people in the world and a billion and 500 million are at risk; these data have urged us to further deepen the topic trying to better clarify the problem.

Of the 700 million person with anemia, 50% are pregnant women, 25% are children, 20% are non-pregnant women and 5% are men.

In athletes and sports people there is an increased percentage of individuals affected by iron deficiency anemia; this fact is found especially in the disciplines of resistance because the continuous sweating facilitates the loss of iron. For this reason those who do amateur or professional sports should consume a greater quantity of foods such as fruits and vegetables that, in addition to bringing the well-known benefits, contain vitamins and all the necessary bio-available iron.

Normally, the iron dose required by the body is assumed thanks to the diet; in meat it is found both iron heme (40%) and non-heme iron (60%), while in plants there is only non-heme iron. The heme iron would seem easier to take, while the non-heme is more sensitive to substances that slow down the absorption (phytates, synthetic vitamins, mineral and ferric supplements, industrial sugars, dairy calcium and derivatives, tea, coffee, smoke, drugs, cocoa and some spices), both to substances that facilitate their absorption.

For optimal iron intake by the body it is necessary the presence of foods containing vitamin C, vitamin E and other organic acids present in fruits, vegetables and sprouts.

The data on the assimilability of iron are very variable and there are no precise values, however we can state that non-heme iron has an assimilability between 2% and 20%, while the absorption of heme iron is about 20%. The daily losses of iron by the body are limited to about 1 mg for men and women in menopause, and 1.5 mg for young women (due to the loss of iron during menstruation); considering the low percentage of absorption, an iron supply of 10 mg for men and 18 mg for women is recommended, while for the daily requirement of pregnancy, the dose rises to 30 mg.

The lower absorption of non-heme iron, compared to the heme, is the basis of the erroneous belief that vegetarians must take at least 1.8 times the amount of iron recommended for meat eaters: this idea, however, has proved inexact in practice. Furthermore, too many iron deposits are a risk factor for many chronic diseases.

Serious iron deficiency can cause anemia, weakness, tachycardia, microcytosis (red blood cells smaller than normal) and worsening of the immune system's function. Excessive presence of iron (possible only through the consumption of meat), however, causes even more serious problems: too much iron deposited in the heart, in the liver and pancreas, causes heart disease, obstruction of arteries with risks of heart attack and stroke, serous, leukocytosis, cirrhosis of the liver and other disorders.

The daily requirement of iron is variable and depends a lot on the different physiological conditions: for example, the regulation of intestinal absorption is fundamental for the balance between income and loss of iron that occur daily in the body. Maintaining the balance of iron in the body depends mainly on the control of absorption of the alimentary iron that takes place in the intestine, especially in the first section (duodenum and jejunum); the absorption of iron decreases when the presence of iron in the body is high, while it increases in the situation of iron deficiency: the more the body needs iron, the greater the intestinal absorption and vice versa.

Beyond a diet poor in iron, there are causes that can cause a reduced absorption, for example: changes in gastric pH (a reduced gastric acid reduces its absorption); substances present in the diet that bind it (reducing the available quota); reduction of the absorbing intestinal surface or alteration of the same; increased intestinal motility; metabolic disorders; Presence of preservatives in foods (EDTA) and substances such as tannates, desalates, phosphates and carbonates.

For very complex physiological reasons, in alcoholics there is often a notable iron deficiency, so those who have iron deficiencies and who like to drink, rather than eat bloody pieces of corpse in quantity, should feed themselves with more natural foods rich in vitamins and pay close attention to the use of alcohol.

Research on the synergies between vitamin C (natural) and its effect in combination with foods rich in iron are numerous; recently these studies have multiplied and their number has made them more independent from the constant supervision of pharmaceutical companies. The analysis carried out by independent scientists regarding food or groups of foods, no longer carried out with the aim of inventing new drugs, have yielded interesting results, with important statistical data concerning the effects on long periods, regarding the consumption of food and their combination.

A research published in the *British Medical Journal* of July 2008 aimed to evaluate the interactions between iron (heme and non heme), red meat, iron supplements and the consequences of these on blood pressure. The study, conducted on 4680 adults between the ages of forty and fifty-nine years, showed that the greater intake of non-heme iron reduces blood pressure; in fact, daily assumptions of non-heme iron, higher than 4.13 mg, were found to be associated with a reduction of 1.45 mmHg of systolic pressure (p <0.001). The intake of heme iron via red meat has instead resulted in a moderate increase in blood pressure: an increase in meat consumption of 103 g in 24 hours has been associated with an increase in systolic pressure of 1.25 mmHg.

In short, this research has shown that consumption of red meat has a negative effect on blood pressure, while the intake of non-heme iron from plants plays a role in preventing and controlling pressure levels.

On April 27 2010, the European Commission requested the Authority for Food Safety (EFSA) to carry out a research to assess the safety of heme iron, when added to food for nutritional purposes as an additional acidce of iron, including supplements.

The group of experts, called by the authorities, after extensive studies has observed that the high intake of heme iron, present in red meat, may be associated with the increased risk of colon cancer. Scientists have concluded that the data in their possession do not allow to demonstrate the safety of the use of heme iron, as an iron acidce for nutritional purposes, and they have stated that iron supplements, red meat and foods with added heme iron, cannot be considered safe for the population.

As already explained in the chapter dedicated to the characteristics of meat, even studies that analyze the consequences of the intake of heme iron have shown a close correlation between the intake of animal products and numerous diseases.

Epidemiological studies on the relationship between diet and health have shown a correlation between the consumption of meat and tumors in the colon, rectum, stomach, pancreas, bladder, ovary, prostate, breast, lung, cardiovascular diseases, rheumatoid arthritis, type two diabetes and Alzheimer's disease.

An umpteenth study carried out in October 2007 and published on the *Medical Hypotheses*, has made clear how the iron of the flesh can harm the organism; vice versa it has emerged that the consumption of non-heme iron of plant origin does not imply any contraindication. The correlation between the emergence of serious diseases and the intake of meat indicates the presence of substances capable of deteriorating important biological contents in the human body. The study was carried out focusing the attention on the oxidative processes deriving from the biochemical processes of heme iron: it has been found that the transformation of iron proteins is contained in raw meat, during its preparation and during its digestion, it generates substances that trigger oxidative reactions.

These reactions damage the lipids, proteins, genetic material, gradually, up to the main organs of the body with an effect similar to that of ionizing radiation. Oxidative damage is widely recognized as one of the causes of the onset of chronic diseases, so it is absolutely clear that reducing the consumption of red meat is essential to avoid the probability of incurring these diseases. Finally, scholars conclude, stating that the intake of fruits and vegetables helps increase the levels of antioxidants in the body, thanks to the presence of selenium, vitamin E, vitamin C, lycopene, cysteine, glutathione and other phytochemicals: all substances capable to counteract the negative effects of oxidative reactions.

It is not the presence of iron in the body that is important for health but its degree of assimilation. The statistics are clear: those who follow a vegan-raw food or frugivorous diet have no deficiencies of any kind, including that relating to iron. The people who have solved the iron deficiency, modifying their diet from omnivorous to raw food, are proof of this.

When the natural diet is followed, the quantity of iron taken is more than sufficient, furthermore its assimilation by the organism is very high.

It is realistically difficult to incur in iron deficiency because the amount of iron present in foods is never the problem, even in cases of large losses due to important periods, pregnancies or intense sports activities. The cause of a possible iron deficiency is not to be found in the quantity of iron taken.

What is compromised, we reiterate, is the assimilative capacity of the organism; to make matters worse, for example, it is dairy products that, besides being iron-free, significantly compromise their absorption. The intestinal villus designed to absorb iron are "covered" by a veil of sticky casein that inhibits its absorbing capacity: dairy products are able to reduce the assimilation of iron even by 50%. This fact greatly limits the ability of the intestine to fulfill its role as an assimilator of useful substances.

Anemic people or those with iron deficiencies should pay more attention to diet and should therefore avoid the substances present in many foods that inhibit iron absorption. These "anti-iron" substances are found in smoking, in drugs, in acidifying meat-based diets, in sugar (even when present in desserts and not only), in salt (and in all salty foods), in supplements, in tea (the tannins present are particularly effective in compromising the absorption of iron), in coffee, in colas, in carbonated drinks, in alcohol, in precooked foods of industrial origin and in boxes in general; moreover phytates present in cereals, phosphates of eggs, soy and its derivatives, whole grains, cabbages - albeit minimally - a cause of poor absorption of iron.

All recent research on the subject, have shown that the best bio-available iron for the human being is that of plant derivation: carrot juice, green leaves, and especially fresh fruit.

What causes anemia is the lack of vitamins C, E, P and an excess of vitamin B12 because it too is in contrast with vitamin C and iron.

The iron that is found in the food is present in the ferric state and to be assimilated must be converted into ferrous form during digestion: the importance of consuming foods rich in vitamin C can be understood well by analyzing this point.

Vitamin C is the greatest architect in the conversion reaction from the ferric to the ferrous state.

We want to reiterate once again an important concept not to be forgotten: the human body can only benefit from the minerals rendered organic by plants, organic minerals that are found only in raw fruits and vegetables because cooking renders inorganic all minerals, therefore no longer assimilable.

The same argument is obviously valid also in reference to the heme iron of animal origin, necessarily consumed after cooking: it is inorganic, therefore not being practically assimilable, it turns out to be only useless and harmful substance that remains in circulation in the organism, doing nothing else that poison it. The same argument also applies to iron that is not present in plants; if you want to obtain all the useful and assimilable nutrients from them, you must necessarily consume them raw.

Let's add a small note regarding Lorenza's personal experience on iron: "*As a child I was very poor in ferritin presenting a hemoglobin with decidedly low values. The doctors suggested to me every time to increase the con-*

sumption of meat and legumes, prescribing iron supplements.

As a good patient I followed all the advice but, while the values of iron and hemoglobin remained very low, I found that the consumption of supplements was due to problems of digestion, liver problems and severe diarrhea. Only after having renounced to follow such advice and after having informed me independently, discovering what is today my diet, I finally managed for the first time to obtain optimal values of ferritin and hemoglobin. For over seven years I have not touched meat and animal products and today all my blood values are perfect. "

In conclusion, as also shown by many statistical data, I can say that it is practically impossible, for those who follow a natural diet, to incur in food shortages of any kind, especially in iron deficiencies, above all because with this diet we assume a much higher amount of vitamin C, compared to any other diet.

16 POLYAMINES

Ever since I was interested in food I tried to find out the truth about the characteristics of food, I found conflicting evidence on everything, except on fruit, the more I insisted on looking for negative factors about fruit and the more we came across positive arguments. Everybody (except for very few exceptions that I will see later) consider fruit an excellent food, even if few know well all the innumerable beneficial characteristics.

If I exclude some variants of macrobiotics which, although without convincing reason, discourage the consumption of fruit, the only apparently unfavorable pretext that I have found concerns *polyamines*.

From my research the polyamine "problem" proved to be non-existent but, having noticed that the topic is rather discussed above online, I decided to make my insights clear.

Polyamine refers to a large category of compounds comprising molecules such as *diamines* (*putrescine* and *cadaverine*), *triamine spermidine* and *tetramine spermine*.

It is not our intention to report in this context the chemical details of these substances, as a summary we can consider that an appropriate definition for polyamine is that of growth regulators since it has been found that some of them play a decisive role in cell growth processes.

These substances are present in many foods such as milk, cheese, cereals, meat and fruit.

Now let's see why the polyamines in fruit (and others) are considered by some to be harmful. According to some research, polyamine, besides being essential molecules for cell growth, could also benefit the growth of cancer cells in cases of existing tumors: the polyamines, acting indiscriminately on each cell, would also promote the growth of those damaged or neoplastic, promoting tumor growth.

The fact that kiwis, oranges and bananas contain discrete doses of polyamine precursors such as *lysine* and *arginine*, has led some researchers to discourage or moderate the consumption of fruit for cancer patients.

The consideration is very strange because the polyamines under accusation are present not only in some fruits but also in corn, meat, milk, cheese, peas, walnuts and, as we have seen, in many other foods.

From a research carried out through a questionnaire on the eating habits of the examined patients, it has been found that an increase in polyamine has a negative effect on colon cancer.

The accuracy of these data seems to us very doubtful, first because the eating habits of the people examined do not mention the percentages of distribution between fruit, meat and other foods, making us suspect that it is not the polyamines present in the fruit that cause growth cancer, but, as now fully demonstrated, it is rather the intake of meat and cheese to cause its development.

Secondly, being the fruit rich in antioxidants and therefore a natural anti-cancer, it cannot be considered a carcinogenic factor under any circumstances, otherwise it would not explain why some alternative fruit-based cancer treatments are so successful.

The studies on polyamines lead researchers to consider an "anti-cancer diet" without products containing polyamines, but this is absolutely irreconcilable with the treatment, since many recommended foods are just the biggest proponents of the carcinogenic processes. Recommending harmful products, just because they are poor in polyamines, is decidedly inconsiderate and, prohibiting the consumption of fruits and vegetables that are rich in phytochemicals and other "anti-cancer" components, seems to us rather ridiculous and dangerous.

I do not want to contest in full the research on polyamines and their pro cancer role, but the problem is that diets are complex: when analyzing the cases according to the diet it is very difficult to blame the single element present in foods, such as polyamines, precisely. It is instead the set of substances taken with the food to cause the many and complex effects on the organism. As I have already amply demonstrated, it is never the single element that causes illness or healing, but rather the context in which it finds itself and the complex synergies with the other substances present in the organism.

These studies have not shown that eating only fruits and vegetables causes an increase in cancer cells, they only found that in some cases, foods containing polyamines taken in a standard diet including meat, milk, fruit, vegetables, cereals, etc., in different percentages, they did not reduce the proliferation of cancer cells.

Some even claim that polyamines could turn into *nitrosamines* (substances produced by intestinal flora starting from nitrites, a type of food additive used as a preservative especially in meat products such as sausages and cured meats), but this would be possible for many other substances: the vitamin C present in vegetables and fruit as well as being an agent that counteracts the carcinogenic activity, is also the substance that blocks the very appearance of the nitrosamines themselves.

The feeling is that after the heme iron, vitamin B12 and Omega-3, polyamines are the new anti-fruit topic now fashionable among those who like to do food terrorism.

I can conclude by declaring that even the "problem" of the polyamines present in the fruit is nothing but a nonsense foolishness from someone who did not want to deepen the subject well.

With this last analysis, regarding the presumed nutritional deficiencies deriving from the fruitarian diet, I have exhausted all the arguments initially perceived as unfavorable. I am sure to have shown the real nutritional characteristics present in fruit.

The science of official nutrition does not set limits on fruit consumption. A concept that I share, even if the limit is in common sense, because eating an exaggerated amount of food although being fruit, is not a healthy attitude.

17 LIMITS OF THE NATURAL DIET

After having dedicated the whole series of books to the exposition of the damage caused by every single food, to praise the greatest benefits of fruit and the advantages, that only a food based nutrition can give, for completeness and honesty, I feel obliged to also expose the limits of such an exclusive diet.

In reality, from a dietary and healthy point of view there are no real limits, it is more a question of psychological and sociological limits. Here, I am not referring to the transition period in which many types of food can still be eaten, therefore remaining within a rather elastic diet, but referring to the "Natural Diet" and the exclusive consumption of fruit.

Regarding the limits due to alleged food shortages, I have already talked about it explaining the groundlessness, now I will discuss the limits from an "existential" point of view.

One of the first concerns regarding our food choice concerns the fact of believing that it is a monotonous and boring diet. Many ask me how I can renounce all the rest, the flavors and the taste of cooked food that seems to be the only reason for life and happiness for the majority of people.

Surely you have asked for it too. I can answer this question only thanks to my experience, to the testimonies and stories of other fruitarians that I have collected in recent years.

There are two types of people who decide to change their diet until they are fed exclusively with fruit. The first, like Lorenza, choose this path driven by real health problems, managing to solve them. The latter, like me, have decided to follow this diet to have a "physical vehicle" of greater performance.

Only those who come to eat only fruit discover that the pleasure and taste that derive from it is so high as to completely forget the previous feelings, deriving from the old diet. In other words, after passing the transition and after a few months of fruition, we no longer feel the necessity, nor the desire, of any other food.

On the contrary, if you try again the old foods after several months, there is a negative sensation on the palate and the taste that once attracted you, now rejects you.

Both those who choose the natural diet by necessity, and those who choose it out of curiosity, for convenience, for radiant health or for other reasons, are often considered by friends, colleagues and relatives as if they had gone out of their mind. This is what has happened to us and sometimes it still happens, even if now we are smiling when we see the expression of incredulity on the part of those who for the first time hear us talking about a natural diet.

The not always positive reactions of friends, relatives, colleagues or spouses can be a negative note because they can easily compromise your new beliefs. In this situation, especially for those who do not live alone, it is necessary to show great willpower; only in this way can one pursue his own path by demonstrating to others the validity of his choices.

I can, in fact, find that friends, colleagues, relatives and all those who a few years ago have seen our diet change, today they show themselves to us much more under- standing; from their face that expression of superiority has disappeared, they have realized that our health has improved considerably, giving us also a better look, they could witness the disappearance of all our health prob- lems and they realized that maybe we are not so crazy, so much that many have started to imitate us.

The second limit of the natural diet is always social, what are we going to do at the restaurant?

Not that dining out is a matter of life or death, but we must admit that in some circumstances it is pleasant and comfortable. Denied forever a dinner with friends or a business lunch could be not only anti-social but, in the long run, even a little sad; as long as you live in this so- ciety it is not always possible to renounce everything, there are situations in which you must or want to take a step back so as not to isolate yourself too much.

When you get used to eating only fruit you do not feel the need for any other food, in fact, as soon as you step out of line, you immediately feel the negative effects in terms of heaviness, drowsiness and much more.

Initially I tried to avoid all situations that included lunch outside the home but today we have partially solved the problem. I do not deny ourselves more to go out with friends in a pizzeria or restaurant to spend an evening in company, I go with them and order what I consider to be the least harmful, for example a mixed salad or a fruit salad; so I do not exclude ourselves from the world and still maintain our diet as much as possible.

I have noticed lately that some restaurants are adapting to the ever increasing demands of vegan and raw food. In fact, many traditional chefs ask us for courses of raw food, so that they can expand their menus by offering their customers more healthy and above all new dishes.

Our opportunities to have lunch or dinner at the restaurant are still limited, therefore, quite irrelevant on our diet, but someone out of necessity could be forced to dine out every day, perhaps eating in the canteen of the company where he works or something else. In these cases, the only solution to continue to follow the fruitarian diet, is to adapt to apples and bananas that are found everywhere or bring the fruit from home.

Lately I have refined my diet by eating both for breakfast and for lunch only apples: these, in addition to making me feel even better, have other practical advantages as apples are easily available, easy to transport, easy to eat and can be kept for long; in the evening, instead, at home and comfortably, I can taste the other types of sweet fruit and indulge ourselves with raw fruitarian recipes with fruits, vegetables and fat fruit.

Eating only apples during the day is very comfortable, we go around a lot and this trick makes our life easier.

However, there are conditions in which to find fruit is not easy, I refer to some excursions in relatively "desert" areas, in the mountains or at the sea; certainly spend one or more weeks on the boat in the middle of the ocean (as we have often done), or go hiking in isolated places lasting a few days, make the supply of fruit quite difficult.

These are exceptional cases that most people will hardly face, but even the most extreme situations can be faced by making an abundant supply of fruit, among which the most comfortable and less perishable are the apples once again or obtaining dried fruits that give a lot of substance, weighs and are not bulky.

It is important not to take everything as a "religion". Even if sometimes you had to eat something else, it should not be considered a drama, as soon as the situation returns to normal, you can start again to follow the natural diet without any problem.

Some say that eating fruit is expensive: it is partially true, fruit today is not particularly cheap especially if you prefer organic products, but apart from those who eat only rice and pasta, on the whole, being fruitarian is no more expensive than being vegan, vegetarian or omnivorous, actually, all things considered, it is also cheaper.

If I then consider that you will no longer use medicines, creams, lotions, eyeglasses, medical examinations, etc., then we can consider, overall, the natural food choice as the least expensive of all, the healthier choice and economic that can be done.

However, I believe that health has no price and, even if eating fruit would be the most expensive choice, it would be the money ever best spent.

I don't find other limits to this diet, the more I think about it, the more positive aspects come to mind. Everyone has their own experiences and points of view, but only after having taken my path you will be able to find only the advantages.

18 CONCLUSIONS ON NATURAL DIET

In this chapter will be exposed the basic concepts of natural diet and further advice on how to apply this diet in the best possible way.

If you have come to read my 4 books until this chapter, you will surely have understood why the fruit is clearly superior to any other food, but you have also read that not all fruit has totally positive characteristics.

In order to get the most out of this diet, we need to know how to create the right pairings, but before explaining in detail the correct combinations between the various types of fruit, I want to reiterate an important concept: to avoid my own mistakes, I suggest, during the food transition, to proceed with a gradual but decisive approach. Only in this way you can get to live on fruit only, avoiding any decompensation and elimination crises, due to a too rapid purification, caused by extremely abrupt dietary changes.

The first thing to do is try to eliminate all junk foods as soon as possible.

If you are still omnivorous you should become a vegetarian, later vegan, then follow a raw food diet, then fruitarians, until you finally reach the natural diet. It is a food path that only you can decide to do, during which you will notice that the closer you are to the natural diet, the more you will notice a clear overall improvement both in terms of physical and psychological health. If you really want to regain real health, you should consider the harmfulness of food, trying to eliminate them according to this order:

Foods like meat, sausages, fish and eggs;

Milk, all dairy products and their derivatives such as cheese, yogurt, ice cream, sweets, etc.;

Honey;

The dried seeds eaten raw like sesame, sunflower, pumpkin, hemp, etc.;

Cooked vegetables;

Cooked cereals including pseudo-cereals;

Oily seeds such as walnuts, almonds, hazelnuts, pine nuts, macadamia, cashews, etc.;

Germinated seeds such as quinoa, amaranth, wheat, etc.;

Plants like mushrooms, shoots, roots, stems, leaves and flowers.

When you come to a fruit-based diet, I recommend eliminating or reducing as soon as possible the acid fruit, then the sweet dried fruit (even if with less urgency).

I can therefore define "the natural diet" a diet comprising dried fruit (not over 42°C or 107°F), fat fruit, sweet fruit and mainly apples: obviously all fresh fruit must be consumed exclusively raw, not frozen and possibly biodynamic or at least biological (however, in the absence of something else, a non-organic fruit is always preferable to any other food, even if of biological origin). Below, I will report the indications on the right combination between the various types of fruit that personally gave my the best results and that I therefore recommend.

I want to remind everyone, regardless of the diet you are currently following, to try to consume as many apples as possible because as I have seen, besides being the favorite fruit, it is also the one that helps the purification process in the most efficient and sweet way, therefore the most suitable for improving or maintaining one's well-being even during a food transition.

I discussed a lot of apples and in this regard I would like to open a parenthesis; there are many people in the world who have been living in perfect health for many years, feeding only with apples. It is not a case, in fact, it is the only food in the world with which you can make a mono-diet and, from a healthy point of view, it is absolutely the best possible food choice.

I understand perfectly how this may seem rather restrictive. I am not proposing you to eat only apples, but it seems right to inform you that it could be a good choice. A diet of only red apples must be achieved very gradually and only after the natural diet pursued by us has been followed for at least a few months.

Let's see now what are the substantial differences between the various fruitarian regimes and the natural diet: although they present minimal differences, they have very different effects, especially in the long term.

The various fruitarian diets that I will analyze, in a short time, might seem already excellent but have some particularities that make them unsustainable for long periods (even for health reasons). On the contrary, the natural diet, if well followed, can be perpetuated with excellent results and without contraindications for an unlimited period.

The so-called *fruitarism* is as old as man. Apparently, our most remote ancestors were born in an optimal environment, where both the climate and the vegetation allowed them to live feeding almost exclusively on fruit, demonstrating excellent health and maximum longevity. This idyllic state lasted about five million years and then, for the now known catastrophic climate disasters that happened about 1.8 million years ago, the human race had to change habits and places; in order to survive, the man adapted himself to eating anything, he began to cultivate, to hunt and to cook foodstuffs, otherwise inedible. Humanity has thus saved itself from extinction, but fell into a pathological state caused by food escamotage that has not yet left. Looking at the relatively recent known history, I have discovered that some ancient language scholars have declared that fruitarianism was a diet, known since more than 4000 years, but due to the difficulty of finding or knowing how to choose the most suitable fruit to man, fruitarianism has never fully developed.

Only a few years ago and thanks also to recent scientific research such as comparative anatomy, comparative phyto-zoological functional morphology, biochemistry and modern nutrition, it has finally come to be established which fruits are truly suitable for human consumption.

If we want, today we have the chance to return to live in perfect health and extreme longevity, just like our ancestors in their best state of millions of years ago.

From the latest scientific research and statistical data collected among fruitarians from all over the world, the real reasons have emerged that have hitherto prevented the development of a healthy and sustainable fruit-based diet; then I analyze what are the negative implications deriving from the wrong choices pursued by almost all the fruitarians of the last millennia.

As a first point, I want to underline that some fruitarians also consume nuts and seeds, therefore, besides not being a "fruitarian diet", it is not even the healthiest choice. With this clarification, I must thoroughly examine the four possible types of fruit-based diets since, it is true that I am evaluating food at the top of the food scale, but if not rightly combined, it can cause some discomfort and becoming, in the long run period, an unsustainable diet.

Here are the combinations to avoid:

First combination: consumption in the same day of both sweet fruit and acid fruit (fresh and dried) and almost no consumption of apples; this combination is usually the most common, especially for those coming from an omnivorous diet.

In the beginning, in fact, we tend to consume fruit with more decisive flavors, just as most of the sweet and acid fruits are. This is because our senses, as well as the taste buds, have been ruined by years of too tasty, too spicy, too sugary and too salty foods, so to appreciate the delicate taste of some fruit, especially apple, it takes the necessary time for taste buds return to their right sensitivity. For this fact, the majority of fruitarians give little consideration to apples and this is a serious mistake.

The sweet fruit is slightly hyperglycaemic and slightly acidifying so it should be balanced by the consumption of some vegetable fruit and fat fruit (which are decidedly alkalizing and partially hypoglycemic).

In this combination, the effects of acid fruit are amplified by consumption of both dried sweet fruit (which is even more hyperglycemic and acidifying than fresh). Increasing the consumption of apples is not decisive, since they are neutral, both from a glycemic and alkalizing point of view; it is for these reasons that eating only with sweet and acid fruit can over time create some disturbances.

I can confirm, by direct experience, that following this type of fruitarianism creates, at least once or twice a week, a strange desire for vegetables, seeds or nuts; these signals are due to the fact that, with this diet, our body feels, sooner or later, the need to counterbalance the effects of sweet fruit and above all of acidity. It is therefore certainly better (also to avoid going back to eating food such as vegetables, which are not fruit), to integrate this diet with vegetable fruit and fat fruit while eliminating the acid one.

Second combination: only fresh and dried sweet fruit.

For the same reasons mentioned above, this choice is not 100% healthy; although excluding acid fruit and increasing the consumption of apples, there remains a certain acidifying and hyperglycemic imbalance.

Third combination: to consume all types of fruit (sweet, acid, vegetable and fat).

In this case, the glycemic and acidifying imbalances caused mainly by the acid and dried sweet fruit, cannot be counterbalanced even by the alkalizing effects of the vegetable and fat fruit.

Fourth combination: only apples, vegetable and fat fruits. In this case, there is a marked decompensation towards too much alkalinity; moreover, fat and vegetable fruits, being hypoglycemic, do not contain enough sugars for the needs of our organism; even if you add to this combination a strong consumption of apples, nothing would be resolved because the apple is already balanced by itself and cannot cover the intake of sugar, lacking in vegetable and fat fruits.

It is therefore necessary the presence of sweet fruit that, with its slight hyperglycemia and acidity, perfectly counterbalances the effects of vegetable and fat fruits.

Of course, the physiological and chemical processes that trigger, according to the various combinations just analyzed, are many and very complex, we avoid reporting them in this context but we can assure you that the final results are exactly those mentioned above.

Our initial mistakes prompted us to personally try all the various combinations of fruit just exposed. So, both because of our direct experience, and the many scientific information learned, especially during these years of research, today we feel honestly ready to show you how to apply the natural diet so you can follow it for as long as you want, obtaining the maximum results.

The Natural diet: in the morning one or two red apples, for lunch at least three types of sweet fruit, according to your fill, and at dinner vegetable and fat fruits (also in the form of raw fruitarian recipes).

When you have arrived at this point, you can take a further step that I have personally considered as the perfect solution, the healthiest, the most comfortable and also the best to maintain the weight: in the morning one or two apples (red), at lunch from three to five apples (possibly red) and at dinner three types of sweet fruit, at will, followed by a plate of vegetable fruit seasoned with avocado, olives (or pitted olive oil) and, finally, a couple of bananas + one apple.

These indications are pretty generic, everyone can vary the quantities according to their needs, the important thing is to keep all the types of fruit reported and consume them in the order indicated.

If you want to maintain maximum physical and mental energy throughout the day, it is important never to reverse what you eat at dinner with what you should eat for lunch.

It may be that some days you are not able to follow these indications to the letter; do not worry, I too cannot always follow them, even if I know that respecting these small rules gives truly surprising results.

I met some people who tried to follow my natural diet but did not succeed, especially for three reasons: they did not follow an adequate transition period, they did a period of fruitarianism without following the right combinations, or they were dissuaded from someone.

As I have already written, very often, especially initially friends and relatives, for various reasons and not always in bad faith, working against, creating a tension that not everyone is able to endure. In this regard, I recommend to all those who want to start this journey, to also involve the people with whom they have more intimate relationships, at least to try to make them understand what it is.

You can justify your choice by having them read this or even other books on this topic. Usually shared knowledge is the key to making social life easier.

Fortunately, many have managed to follow the natural diet correctly, with a minimum of commitment, especially initial.

Thus they entered an unknown world that gave them health and joy of life. They finally discovered all the fantastic sensations arising from eating only fruit and today they do not want to go back.

Each of you will have to follow the instinct, pursuing your choice, whatever it is, with confidence and conviction.

Surely it will be the best change you can take in your life. Do not worry too much, know that changing old eating habits is much easier than you can imagine, it is only a matter of starting gradually and, little by little, you will be projected into a world where there are no limits.

FINAL CONCLUSIONS

"Do not believe in something, just because it has been reported to you, do not believe in traditions handed

*down from antiquity, nor in gossip as such, nor in the
writings of wise men, just because composed by them, or
in the fantasy we suspect may have been stimulated by
some divinity, neither in the inferences originated by
random assumptions, neither in what appears to be an
analogical necessity, nor in the mere authority of teach-
ers and superiors. Believe only when writings, doctrines
or sayings are corroborated by
your reason and awareness "*
(Gautama Buddha)

Deep and intelligent words I have decided to report because, in addition to sharing them fully, I consider them
perfect for evaluating the contents of this series of
books.

I have done my best to try to inform you about the very
close relationship between food and health, but my work
is over.

From today and throughout the rest of your life, your
well-being and therefore your happiness will depend
only on your future food choices.

Good health to everyone.

Diego Pagani

If you have not read the other 3 books of the "*How to find health*" series, click here: https://goo.gl/yQbj1E

www.howfindhealth.com

"Tell The World What You Think Of This Book.
Would you mind taking a few seconds
to leave an honest review?
It's important because your opinion
helps people make better decisions."

Diego Pagani

Bibliography

Author	Title	Year	Edition
Ehret, Arnold	*Prof. Arnold Ehret's Mucusless Diet Healing System*	1924	Ehret Literature
Peter Jentschura	la salute attraverso eliminazione delle scorie	2006	Jentschura Verlag
Harvey e Marlin Diamond	A tutta salute	1989	Sperling & Kupfer S.p.A.
A.M. King	io sono immortale	2010	Io sono Edizioni
4	la vita segreta delle piante		
Max Gerson	Gerson Therapy Handbook	1999	Gerson Institute
Edmond Bordeaux Szekely	il vangelo esseno	2006	manca edizioni
norman walker	Succhi Freschi di Frutta e Verdura	2012	Macro edizioni
Deepak Chopra	Corpo senza eta mente senza tempo	2005	Sperling & Kupfer S.p.A.
Herbert M. Shelton	il digiuno puo salvarvi la vita	1986	Società Editrice Igiene Naturale s.r.l.

William Dufty	Sugar Blues	2005	Macro edizioni
T. Colin Campbell	The China study	2011	Macro edizioni
Anatomia Umana	Paolo Castano, Lucio Cocco, Alessandra De Barbieri, Loredana D'Este, Francesca Floriani, Gherardo Gheri, Maria Rita Mondello, Stefano Papa, Pietro Petriglieri, Giuliano Pizzini, Carlo Ridola, Stelio Rossi, Giovanni Sacchi, Paola Sirigu, Salvatore Spinella	2003	edi-ermes
Renzo Minelli	Appunti di fisiologia umana. Programma per la tabella XVIII, fisiologia della respirazione e dell'equilibrio acido base	2013	Editore Medea
B. B. Buchanan	Biochimica e biologia molecolare delle piante	2003	Zanichelli
Reginald H. Garrett	Reginald H. Garrett	2008	Zanichelli
Graham Hancock	Impronte degli dei	1992	TEA
Graham Hancock	Talismano. Le città sacre e la Fede segreta	2004	TEA

Henry Gray	Anatomy of the human body	1918	*Lea & Febiger*
Frank H. Netter,	*Atlante di anatomia umana, 3ª edizione*	2007	*Elsevier Masson*
Zaccaria Fumagalli	*Anatomia umana normale*	1983	Piccin
Dee Unglaub Silverthorn	*Fisiologia umana*	2010	*Pearson Education Italia*
Luigi Grazioli, Lucio Olivetti	*Diagnostica per immagini delle malattie del fegato e delle vie biliari*	2005	*Elsevier*
Charles A. Janeway, Paul Travers, Mark Walport, Mark J. Shlomchik	*Immunobiologia (3ª edizione italiana sulla 6ª inglese)*	2007	Piccin
Giuliano Ricciotti	*Biochimica di base*	2008	*Italo Bovolenta*
V. Donald, Voet Judith G. e Pratt Charlotte W	*Fondamenti di biochimica,*	2001	Zanichelli
Berg Jeremy M., Tymoczko John L. e Stryer Lubert	*Biochimica*	2003	Zanichelli
H. J. M. Bowen	*Trace Elements in Biochemistry*	1976	Academic Press

Carlo M. Rotella, Edoardo Mannucci, Barbara Cresci	*Criteri diagnostici e* terapia	1999	*S E E Editrice* Firenze
Giovanni Faglia, Paolo Beck- Peccoz	*del sistema endocrino e del metabolismo 4ª* edizione	2006	*McGraw-* Hill
R e s e a r c h Laboratories Merck	*Merck Manual quinta* edizione	2008	Springer-Verlag
Gremigni P, Letizia L	*Il problema obesità. Manuale per tutti i professionisti della* salute	2011	*Maggioli* Editore
William E. Winter, Maria *R i t a* Signorino, Diabe tes Mellitus	*Pathophysiology, E t i o l o g i e s , C o m p l i c a t i o n s , M a n a g e m e n t , and* Laboratory Evaluation	####	Assoc. for *C l i n i c a l* Chemistry
F u m e n t o , Michael	*The Fat of the Land:* Our Health Crises and *H o w O v e r w e i g h t* Americans can Help Themselves	1997	*P e n g u i n* Books
Keller, Kathleen	E n c y c l o p e d i a o f Obesity	2008	*S a g e* Publicatio ns, Inc
K o l a t a , Gina, Rethinkin g Thin	*new science of weight loss - and the myths and realities of dieting*	2007	Picador
Levy-Navarro, Elena	*The Culture of Obesity in Early and Late* Modernity	2008	*Palgrave* Macmillan

) Pool, Robert, Fat	Fighting the Obesity Epidemic	2001	Oxford, UK
M. Wabitsch, J. Hebebrand, W. Kiess, K. Zwiauer	Child and Adolescent Obesity: Causes and Consequences, Prevention and Management	2004	Springer
M. Wabitsch, J. Hebebrand, W. Kiess, K. Zwiauer	Child and Adolescent Obesity	2005	Piper
Manzi G	L'evoluzione umana. Ominidi e uomini prima di Homo sapiens	2007	Il Mulino
Hermann Bengtson	Introduction to Ancient History	1975	University of California Press
Hulda Regehr Clark	The Cure for All Cancers	1993	New Century Press
Alex Jack	Il cibo medicina	2005	Hermes
Bates Williams	Vista perfetta senza occhiali - ebook	2014	Loredana de Michelis
Wilson Lawrence	Equilibrio nutrizionale e analisi minerale tessutale		Sinai Edizioni
Rothwell NJ, Stock MJ	Influence of carbohydrate and fat intake on diet-inuduced thermobenesis and brown fat activity	1987	J Nutr 117

Stirling Jl, Stock MJ	Metabolic originis of thermogenesis by diet	1968	nature 200
Horio F, Youngman LD, Bell RC	Thermogenesis, low-protein diets and decresed development of AFB1-induced preneoplastic foci in rat liver	1991	Nutr Cancer 16
Youngman LD	The growth and development of aflatoxin B1-induced preneoplastic lesion, tumors, metastasis and spontaneous tumors as they are influence by dietary protein level.	1990	Ph.D Thesis 1990
Robbins J.	The food Revolution	2001	Barkeky, CA
Macilwain G.	The general nature and treatment of Tumors	1845	John Churchill
Associated press	Survey: many guidelines qritten by doctor with ties to companies	2002	The Itaca Journal 12 Feb
Olivieri NF	Patients' health or company profits? The commercialization of academy reserch.	2003	Engineering Ethics
Chopra SS	Industry funding of clinical trials: benefict or bias?	2003	Jama 290

Moyniham R.	Who pays dor the pizza? Redefining the relationships between doctor and drug company	2003	Brit. Med. Journal 326
Eberhardt MV, Lee CY, Liu RH	Antioxidant activity of fresh apples	2000	Nature 405
Boseley S.	Sugar industry threatens to scupper WHO	2003	The Guardian 21 April
Albert CM, Hennekens CH, O'Donnell CJ	Fish consumption and risk of sudden cardiac death	1998	Jama 289
Informatio Plus	Nutrition a key to good health	1999	informatio n Plus
Valdo Vaccaro	Alimentazione Naturale - Vol. 2 - Libro	2014	Anima Edizioni
Valdo Vaccaro	Alimentazione Naturale - Vol.1- Libro	2009	Anima Edizioni
Giovannucci E, Rimm E Liu Y	A prospective study of tomato product, lycopene and prostate cancer risk	2002	Nat. Cancer Institute
Yaukey J	Changing cows diests elevates milks' caner.fighting	1996	Ithaca Journal
Joel Fuhrman	Eat to Live: The Amazing Nutrient-Rich Program for Fast and Sustained Weight Loss, Revised Edition	2011	Little brown and company

Lorenzo Acerra	Il Mal di Latte Il Mal di Latte Intolleranze,allergie e malattie da latte e latticini	2008	Macro Edizioni
Frank A. Oski	Don't Drink Your Milk!	1992	Teach Services Inc
Matthew D. Warner	Fruitarians Are The Future	2012	Independent Publishing Platform
Douglas N. Graham	The 80/10/10 Diet	2006	FoodnSport Press
Jesse J Jacoby	The Raw Cure: Healing Beyond Medicine: How self-empowerment, a raw vegan diet, and change of lifestyle can free us from sickness and disease	2012	SoulSpire
Ralph E Phd Carson	Harnessing The Healing Power Of Fruit: The New Paradigm for Optimum Health	2009	Siloam
Anne Osborne	Fruitarianism : The Path To Paradise	2009	Anne Osborne; Third Printing
Robert S. Morse N.D	The Detox Miracle Acidcebook: Raw Food and Herbs for Complete Cellular Regeneration	2004	Kalindi Press

norman walker	la salute dell'intestino	2012	Macro edizioni
Herbert M. Shelton	Food Combining Made Easy	2012	Book Pub Company; 3rd edition
Herbert M. Shelton	The History of Natural Hygiene and Principles of Natural Hygiene	2010	Kessinger Publishing, LLC
Keith Woodford	Devil in the Milk: Illness, Health and the Politics of A1 and A2 Milk	2009	Chelsea Green Publishing

"How to find health" serie:

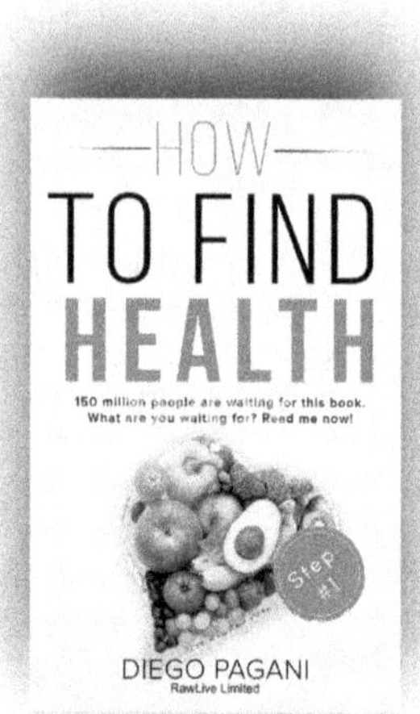 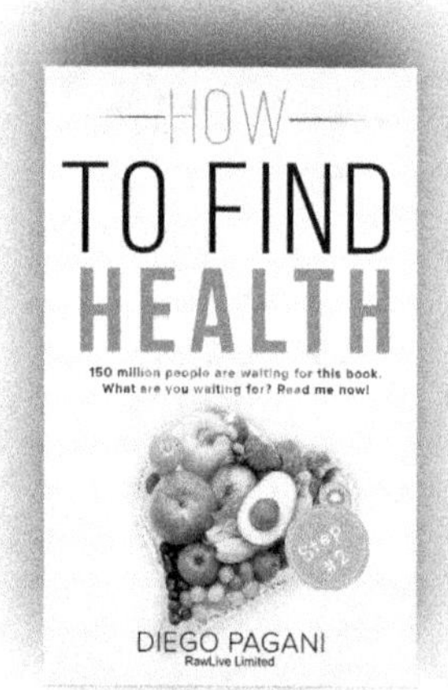

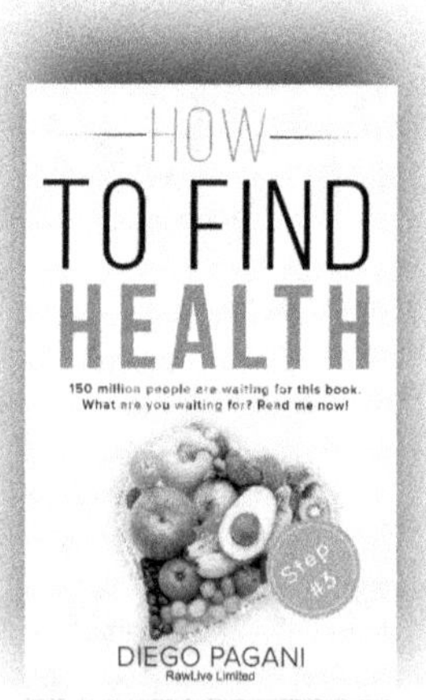 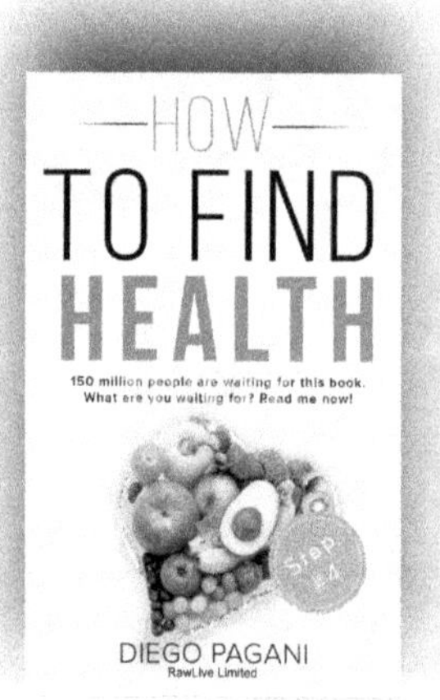

www.howfindhealth.com